Homelessness and Social Policy

Edited by Roger Burrows, Nicholas Pleace and Deborah Quilgars

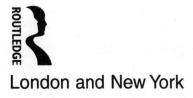

London and New York

First published 1997 by Routledge
11 New Fetter Lane, London EC4P 4EE

Simultaneously published in the USA and Canada
by Routledge
29 West 35th Street, New York, NY 10001

Typeset in Times by
J&L Composition Ltd, Filey, North Yorkshire
Printed in Great Britain by Hartnolls Ltd., Bodmin, Cornwall

British Library Cataloguing in Publication Data
A catalogue record for this book is available from the British
Library

Library of Congress Cataloging in Publication Data
Homelessness and social policy/edited by Roger Burrows,
    Nicholas Pleace, and Deborah Quilgars.
        p.   cm.
Includes bibliographical references and index.
    1. Homelessness—Great Britain. 2. Homeless
persons—Government policy—Great Britain. I. Burrows,
Roger, 1962– . II. Pleace, Nicholas, 1965– .
III. Quilgars, Deborah, 1965– .
HV4545.A4H66 1997   97–2330
362.5′8′0941–dc21   CIP

ISBN 0–415–15456–1 (hbk)
ISBN 0–415–15457–X (pbk)

Contents

List of tables

Notes on contributors

Isobel Anderson is currently a lecturer in the Housing Policy and Practice Unit at the University of Stirling. She was previously a research fellow in the Centre for Housing Policy at the University of York.

Mark Bevan is currently a researcher in the Department of Town and Country Planning at the University of Newcastle upon Tyne. He was previously a research fellow in the Centre for Housing Policy at the University of York.

Wendy Bines is currently working in the NHS. She was previously a research fellow in both the Social Policy Research Unit and the Centre for Housing Policy at the University of York.

Roger Burrows is Assistant Director of the Centre for Housing Policy at the University of York.

Jane Carlisle is currently a postgraduate student at the University of York. She was previously a research fellow in the Centre for Housing Policy at the University of York.

Janet Ford is Director of the Centre for Housing Policy at the University of York and holds the Joseph Rowntree Foundation Chair in Housing Policy.

John Greve is an associate of the Centre for Housing Policy at the University of York. He was previously Professor of Social Administration at the University of Leeds. He is the author of classic studies of homelessness in the 1960s, 1970s and 1980s.

Paul Higate is currently a postgraduate student at the University of York.

Peter A. Kemp is Professor of Housing and Urban Studies and Director of the ESRC Centre for Housing Research and Urban Studies at the University of Glasgow. He was previously the first Joseph Rowntree Professor of Housing Policy and founding Director of the Centre for Housing Policy at the University of York.

Stuart Lowe is a lecturer in the Department of Social Policy and Social Work and an associate of the Centre for Housing Policy at the University of York.

Joanne Neale is currently a research fellow in the Centre for Drug Misuse Research at the University of Glasgow. She was previously a postgraduate student in the Centre for Housing Policy at the University of York.

Christine Oldman is a research fellow in the Centre for Housing Policy at the University of York.

Nicholas Pleace is a research fellow in the Centre for Housing Policy at the University of York.

Deborah Quilgars is a research fellow in the Centre for Housing Policy at the University of York.

David Rhodes is a research fellow in the Centre for Housing Policy at the University of York.

Julie Rugg is a research fellow in the Centre for Housing Policy at the University of York.

Preface
Homelessness then and now

John Greve

Homelessness in Britain is not a recent phenomenon. There has always been a substantial minority of people who, for a variety of reasons, have been unable to provide or retain housing for themselves or their families. The patterns of causes have changed over time, but poverty has persisted as a key factor.

For centuries a major responsibility of the parishes and, later, the Poor Law system, was to provide shelter for homeless people. This responsibility was transferred to the new local authority welfare departments in 1948. Significantly, the duties and powers of these departments were defined by the National Assistance Act 1948, which inherited and perpetuated much of the philosophy and some of the practices of the hated Poor Law (see Chapter 2, this volume, for a more detailed account).

It was not until 1977 that local authority housing departments were given explicit responsibility for rehousing those homeless families and individuals who, after assessment, were deemed to have met the statutory criteria for determining whether or not they were homeless (see Chapter 1, this volume, which also considers how homelessness has been defined).

There was a sudden flood of homelessness after the war, from 1947 to 1951, notably in London. The causes were associated with the war and the widespread confusions and dislocations created by the attempts to adjust rapidly to peacetime conditions. Feelings of disappointment and resentment swelled, and the 'squatting' of unoccupied buildings spread swiftly. It was to recur twenty years later, again as a response to rising homelessness.

During the war, house building had ceased almost totally for five years, while hundreds of thousands of houses had been destroyed or made uninhabitable by bombing. Others had become unfit through neglect and lack of maintenance or repair. After the war, millions of people were demobilised from the Armed Forces or war work and, together with evacuees, returned to their home areas. Marriages boomed and the birth rate accelerated.

By the early 1950s new building and the repairs programme were making substantial inroads into some of the most acute shortages of accommodation, but sharing was very widespread – and was accepted as a normal feature of homemaking. Family homelessness, however, was still a significant problem, especially in London, and council-house waiting lists were lengthening in all parts of the country. During this first post-war period, 80 per cent or more of all house building was for local councils, and all use of building materials and labour was tightly controlled, as were rents and expenditure on construction and repairs. Meanwhile, it was not uncommon for young families to have to face ten years or longer on the waiting list.

In the late 1950s and, more obviously in the early 1960s, a marked and, as it proved, continuous increase in homelessness became apparent – first, and most substantially, in London but later in other parts of the country. The increase was most evident in major urban centres which, like London and Birmingham, were experiencing rapid economic growth accompanied by an expansion in white-collar and professional occupations, all of which exerted severe pressure on the housing markets (Greve 1964; Greve *et al.* 1971).

As the 1960s progressed, observers began to identify the characteristics of a national problem emerging from what had hitherto been perceived by many – not least in government circles – as local, transient, marginal, and mainly affecting 'problem families' (Glastonbury 1971).

Homelessness in London attracted greatest attention from the media, politicians and the public – mainly because of its scale and visibility. But, since the 1960s, homelessness outside the capital has increased faster than in London.

From the 1960s to around 1990, the numbers of people accepted annually as homeless by local authorities in Britain multiplied between ten- and twentyfold, depending on the type of area (Greve 1991). The average annual rate of increase in homelessness for England as a whole was about 50 per cent higher than for London, and higher still in some local authority areas. By 1990, nearly four-fifths of households accepted as homeless by local authorities in Britain were recorded outside London.

In the 1960s and early 1970s homelessness was still seen as predominantly a London problem and caused by the unique characteristics of the metropolis. By the end of the 1980s, the picture had been transformed. Homelessness can now be seen to be a problem affecting different kinds of area, from crowded inner-city conurbations to picturesque rural villages, and involving a wider spectrum of population (Greve 1991). Its roots have spread widely and deeply into the social fabric.

Numbers

The number of people who have experienced homelessness is very large, Greve (1991) calculated that in the decade up to 1990 over one million households – around three million people – in Britain were accepted by local authorities on grounds of homelessness. This is consistent with later figures reported in this volume showing that, in England alone, 1.42 million households were accepted by local authorities as 'statutorily homeless' between 1984 and 1995.

In the period 1959–60, the numbers of households admitted to temporary or short-stay accommodation by local authorities, in any one year, amounted in total to a few thousand, the great majority in London. But the numbers rose with remarkable consistency from the early 1960s – and spread geographically, as has been mentioned. In 1995, the peak year, local councils in England accepted nearly 145,000 households as 'statutorily homeless', the great majority of them families, but including thousands of individual persons. To view the incidence of homelessness from another perspective: one of the studies discussed in the present volume (Chapter 4) found that 4.3 per cent of a large sample of heads of household reported that they had been homeless at some time in the previous ten years.

It should be noted that most of the figures referring to homelessness, which have been cited above, apply to homeless families or to individuals accepted by local authorities as coming into priority categories in relation to homelessness. The extent of homelessness among lone persons or families without dependent children is heavily understated by relying on local authority returns alone.

Some comparisons over time

It is possible to make some broad comparisons of survey findings on homelessness over the past four decades. The sources of information for these comparisons are: studies of homelessness in London carried out in 1961–62 (Greve 1964) and 1969–70 (Greve *et al.* 1971), a wider study of homelessness in Britain (Greve 1991), and the detailed investigations of different aspects of homelessness discussed in the chapters of the present book.

Causes of homelessness

The two earlier studies referred to above (1961–62 and 1969–70) were concerned with London – in the first, the London County Council area, broadly the Inner London of the reformed post-1964 system; and Greater London in the second study. The most important immediate causes of homelessness identified in 1970 were much the same as in 1959–60: relationship breakdown; landlords requiring the accommodation (including eviction); and rent arrears in private or local authority housing. Other significant causes mentioned were: overcrowding; harassment by landlords; and unauthorised occupancy of a council dwelling. Mortgage arrears were mentioned by only about 1 per cent of homeless households in 1959–60. This remained a relatively insignificant cause of homelessness at the end of the 1960s, but emerged as a significant factor in the late 1980s and early 1990s (Chapter 6, this volume).

By the late 1980s, and viewing Britain as a whole, the most important immediate causes of homelessness showed some change by comparison with 1959–60 and 1969–70. Most prominent now were (still) the breakdown of relationships (including those between young people and their parents or guardians), the failure of sharing arrangements in accommodation and unemployment. The first two factors had remained important over the thirty years or so up to 1990 and continue to be so. Unemployment increased in importance as a cause from the 1960s onwards. At the beginning of the 1960s one in ten of the men admitted by local authorities, with their families, to temporary accommodation in London was unemployed. By 1969, the proportion had trebled to 30 per cent, and a large number of those not actually unemployed at the time of admission had a history of unstable employment. Since then, unemployment has persisted as a major contributory factor associated with homelessness.

Income

Throughout all the studies, the households and individuals accepted by local authorities – whether in London or other parts of Britain –

have been predominantly on low incomes. In the early 1960s this usually meant low, but often intermittent, income from employment – in early 1962 unemployment benefit provided the income for one in ten of the men admitted to homeless accommodation in London County, while a similar proportion of families were dependent on National Assistance Benefits (Greve 1964). As time went on, unemployment and dependency on social security benefits came to figure increasingly large among the homeless population.

Marital status

Lone parents with dependent children are particularly at risk of homelessness, as numerous studies – including those considered in this volume – have shown. Statistically, lone parent families who become homeless are over represented about tenfold by comparison with their numbers in the general population. Evidence for the growth of this problem was already discernible in the late 1950s and early 1960s. The London study of 1961–62 found that 41 per cent of the women who were admitted to temporary accommodation with their children were separated (29 per cent), divorced (2 per cent) or single (9 per cent). The proportions for 1966–69 were much the same, but with relatively fewer separated (25 per cent), and more single parents (12 per cent). But in all categories, the absolute numbers were much greater, and continued to rise until the early 1990s.

Age

Consistently, since the late 1950s, the majority of women with children accepted by local authorities as homeless have been under the age of thirty, with about half of these under the age of twenty-five, and a substantial percentage under twenty years old. There has been a tendency for the average age of women admitted to fall at the same time as the number of homeless families accepted by local authorities has increased (up to recent years).

Children

Although the majority of families with children accepted by local authorities as homeless do not differ greatly from the average family in Britain, in terms of the numbers of children, larger families do tend to be over represented. Nevertheless, over the past thirty-five years and more, most homeless families have had one or two children. In 1959, 71 per cent of admissions in London were in that category, in the period 1966–69 it had fallen to 54 per cent of the total, while families with four or more children had risen from 14 per cent in 1959 to 25 per cent in 1966–69. In the 1966–69 period, families with four or more children were three times as common among homeless admissions as they were among all London families.

Young lone mothers, and larger-than-average families with dependent children, have continued to be over-represented among the homeless. In terms of numbers, this is particularly true of lone parent families. Typically, these characteristics are linked with low income and reliance on social security benefits, and this compounds their vulnerability in the housing market.

Place of birth·

Accurate information on ethnicity was not available to the London studies of 1961–62 or 1969–70, but data on place of birth throw some light on ethnic origins. Until the last quarter of 1969 fewer than one homeless adult in fifty among those admitted to temporary accommodation in London County was born in a Commonwealth country or 'other overseas territory'. Meanwhile, up to a fifth had been born in Eire. By 1969, the number of applicants to local authorities in Greater London – a much larger area than in the 1961–62 survey, had increased very considerably, and the pattern had changed in significant ways. The proportion of Irish-born had fallen by more than half to 7.6 per cent – though overall numbers had risen – while the percentage of Commonwealth-born (mostly Caribbean, according to other sources) had multiplied fifteenfold to over 30 per cent. Again, the absolute numbers had also multiplied. The total number of people in temporary accommodation in Inner London more than trebled between 1960 and 1970 and had grown even faster in Outer London (Greve *et al.* 1971).

The surge in homelessness among ethnic-minority groups (including those of Irish descent), which began in the early 1960s, became a major feature of homelessness. They are heavily over-represented among homeless families – and, not least, young single persons – in London and larger urban areas outside the capital. Homelessness is a particularly acute problem in places such as Inner London and comparable areas in other conurbations, which are also concentrations of housing stress. In such areas, the interaction between unemployment, vulnerability and homelessness are particularly strong.

The aim of this preface has been to take a brief look back at some of the features of homelessness, as they have evolved over nearly four decades. The chapters of the main volume examine in detail a variety of aspects and perspectives of homelessness within the contemporary period.

Acknowledgements

Thanks are due to Jane Allen, Susan Anscombe, Joanne Gatenby and Margaret Johnson for their administrative assistance in all of the research reported in this volume. Thanks are also due to all of the people who have, at various times, participated in the various research projects which provide the basis for many of the chapters.

Chapter 1

Homelessness in contemporary Britain
Conceptualisation and measurement

Nicholas Pleace, Roger Burrows and Deborah Quilgars

This book is about homelessness and social policy in contemporary Britain. It brings together in one place a range of conceptual and empirical studies of various aspects of homelessness which have been carried out by researchers at the Centre for Housing Policy (CHP) at the University of York throughout the 1990s.[1] This opening chapter attempts to define what is meant by homelessness and how the phenomena might be measured. It also provides a brief summary of the structure of the rest of the book.

WHAT IS HOMELESSNESS?

In the United Kingdom homelessness has come to be defined and discussed in terms of the main policy response to the problem. This policy response was the 1977 Housing (Homeless Persons) Act that for the first time placed duties on local authority housing departments not only to rehouse homeless individuals and families permanently, but to do so as a matter of priority. The basic legislation passed unaltered into the 1985 Housing Act until it was replaced with new legislation within the 1996 Housing Act, see Lowe (this volume) for detailed discussion.[2]

Until the 1977 Act, responses from the then Department of Health and Social Security (DHSS) and local social services departments retained many similarities to Victorian responses to extreme poverty. Gender separation of homeless families to fit them into traditional hostel accommodation was common practice, and as late as 1974/75, 2,800 children were placed in care merely because their families had been found homeless by local authorities (Richards 1993). The reasons for such harsh policy responses were largely underpinned by the dominance of political ideologies which emphasised individual responsibility over structural causes and, relatedly, made clear distinctions between the 'deserving' and the 'undeserving' (Lowe, this volume; Neale, this volume). Within such a dominant conceptual frame people who became homeless were often considered to be responsible for their own plight because they were choosing not to work, refusing responsibility or because they were 'drunkards'. For example, when the first legislation to provide assistance to homeless people was being debated in 1977, they were described as 'queue jumpers, rent dodgers, scroungers and scrimshankers' by a Conservative MP speaking for the then largely Conservative Association of District Councils (Richards 1993). Hesitancy about the adequacy of explanations of homelessness which relied upon people supposedly deliberately *choosing* to be homeless only began in the late 1960s – well behind the acceptance of structural explanations of other social issues and problems. The health problems and drug and alcohol dependency of many single homeless people were recorded, and studies began to identify the role of housing supply, relationship breakdown and economic change in the production of homelessness more generally.

For several years, some studies placed emphasis on structural causes of *single* homelessness (mainly housing supply) (Drake *et al.* 1982) while other studies, particularly in the United States, identified mental health problems as the underlying cause of single homelessness (Basuk 1984). It was only relatively recently that more sophisticated research began to appear that advanced the argument that single homelessness was caused by social and economic changes which disproportionately affected the most vulnerable in society (Caton 1990; Dant and Deacon 1989). The same kind of debate never existed in relation to *homeless families*, who were from the 1970s in the United Kingdom much more likely to be seen as victims of circumstance (Glastonbury 1971). There was also less debate about whether the state should intervene because children, who were almost universally accepted as being unable to help themselves, were present in homeless families.

The 1977 and 1985 Acts represent a policy response caught between the movement away from the more primitive 'explanations' of homelessness and towards explanations more firmly rooted in research. On one level, the 1977 Act recognised homelessness as a structural phenomenon by addressing the problem with the provision of housing for families, couples and individuals who became homeless. However, because the 1977 Act was passed at a time when the older 'explanation' of homelessness as an individual choice still held some sway, it still contains strong residual elements which reflect this. Essentially, the Act could not go all the way in accepting that social and economic factors were largely to blame for homelessness because the popular conception of 'scroungers' was still too strong. The Act therefore divided the homeless population of the United Kingdom into homeless people who could not help their situation and should be helped, while refusing assistance to people who could 'help themselves'. Thus the Act (re)created *deserving* homeless people (homeless families and very vulnerable single people) who could receive assistance under the Act, and *undeserving* homeless people (lone homeless people and couples without serious illness or impairment) who must be refused such assistance.

Of course, any government is always concerned to keep expenditure down and rationing services on some basis is always necessary. However, while access to other welfare services is relatively simple – one must demonstrate unemployment to get benefit, present with a health problem to get NHS services and so forth – access to assistance if one is homeless is not just a question of proving that one is homeless. Homeless people must show that they have not made themselves homeless on purpose (called 'intentionally homeless') and they must usually prove a 'local connection' to the housing authority to which they are applying for assistance. It must also be clear that they have not left any accommodation that they could reasonably be expected to occupy. Once all that has been proven, a homeless person must also demonstrate that they are a member of one of the 'deserving' groups of homeless people, whom the 1985 Act and code of guidance says can receive assistance, referred to as being in a situation of *priority need*:

- those who are pregnant, or who live in a household with someone who is pregnant;
- those who live in a household that contains one or more dependent children; and
- those who live in a household that contains a person who is vulnerable under the terms of the code of guidance to the 1985 Housing Act.

Those who are vulnerable include:

- people who find it difficult to fend for themselves due to old age;
- people with learning difficulties;
- people with a mental health problem;

- disabled people; and
- people who are vulnerable for 'other special reasons'.

These 'other special reasons' include:

- children and women who are escaping violence or abuse;
- people escaping racial abuse; and
- young people considered to be at risk.

Some authorities have interpreted this duty as including people with drug and/or alcohol dependencies, certain categories of ex-offender and people with terminal or life-threatening illnesses such as HIV/AIDS.

These categories appear to be substantially unaltered in the 1996 Housing Act (Section 189), although the detailed guidance to the new Act had not yet been released at the time of writing. Recent amendments to the 1985 Housing Act, which are also present in the 1996 Act, prevent asylum seekers from getting assistance from local authorities under the homelessness legislation. Once accepted under the 1977 and 1985 Acts, homeless people had priority access to permanent rehousing in local authority or housing association stock – although a few authorities had also started to use the private rented sector (PRS) by the mid-1990s, raising debates about what exactly 'permanent' meant. The 1996 Housing Act will introduce an *interim duty to accommodate* statutorily homeless households for up to two years (Section 192) while they join the waiting list with everyone else who is seeking a council or housing association home. This change, it was argued by the government, would increase the fairness of the allocation of social housing (Bevan and Rhodes, this volume; Lowe, this volume).

Homelessness is described in the United Kingdom along the lines of the homelessness legislation. *Non-statutory homeless* people are those who cannot get access to accommodation because they fall outside the groups specified by the 1977, 1985 and 1996 Acts. This group is largely made of single people without children who do not qualify for assistance because they are not 'vulnerable' under the terms of the legislation and are generally called *single homeless people* (Kemp, this volume). Those who qualify for assistance are called *statutorily homeless people*.

These definitions are not clear cut, mainly because local authorities have considerable discretion in the interpretation of the code of guidance to the 1985 Act (something that will probably be true of the 1996 Act too) and varying capacities, in terms of available stock, to respond to the needs of homeless people. Acceptance as statutorily homeless by a local authority in one area does not mean that another authority would also accept one as homeless (Niner 1989; Butler *et al.* 1994). It is possible to argue that those who are placed in the worst position by the resource limitations of local authorities are single homeless people, since the severity or presence of an Act-defined 'vulnerability' is debatable, while the presence of a child or signs of pregnancy are not (Pleace and Quilgars 1996).

In addition, acceptance as homeless under the Act may not mean that homelessness is going to end immediately. In some (though not all) areas, pressure on the council and housing association stock is such, with an average wait of 1.9 years on the waiting list for non-homeless people seeking rehousing (Prescott-Clarke *et al.* 1994, para 5.7.1), that statutorily homeless people have sometimes to wait many months or even years in temporary accommodation and remain, in effect, homeless. When the 1996 Housing Act comes into effect, all statutorily homeless people will remain in this state of effective homelessness for up to two years before they are permanently rehoused (Bevan and Rhodes, this volume; Lowe, this volume).

The homelessness legislation, while to a limited extent representing a progression in 1977 because of the duties to provide housing to women escaping violence, was not designed with the needs of women in mind. The focus was on homeless families and homeless single men, rather than on the specific needs of women (Neale, this volume; Watson and Austerberry 1986) – a situation that has not changed with the introduction of the 1996 Housing Act.

Within the single homeless population, there are subdivisions. Many single homeless people are in some form of accommodation, particularly if they fall into the groups to which charitable and voluntary groups provide services. Many organisations, including local authorities and housing associations, provide hostels or day centres for single homeless people, who are a mainly male population, and there are also many organisations focusing on young people who are homeless. The bulk of the non-statutorily homeless population is in some form of accommodation, though not in housing, for much of the time because of this provision. However, there is also a (probably) much smaller population of *people sleeping rough*, who sleep outside for some or all the time. This group, characterised by very poor health status (Bines, this volume; Pleace and Quilgars, this volume) are those who perhaps more than any other group represent the popular conception of homelessness.

Research (Kemp, this volume; Randall and Brown 1993) has shown that the needs of single homeless people and people sleeping rough are often as great as those of statutorily homeless people. Campaigning organisations, such as Campaign for the Homeless and Roofless (CHAR), argue that the distinction in the 1985 Act is artificial and that many single homeless people require assistance and, relatively frequently, care and support services. Recent government responses, including the *Rough Sleepers Initiative* (RSI) and the *Homelessness Mentally Ill Initiative* have tacitly accepted this basic argument. In effect, it could be argued that there is a recognition in the RSI, which is now in its third phase (extending outside London for the first time), that the policy response that should be dealing with the needs of homeless people who require assistance, the 1985 Act, was not working properly.

It is possible then to generate the following classification of homelessness in the United Kingdom. However, it is important to bear in mind that each group has 'fuzzy' edges because the policy response and service provision vary between different areas.

1 *Statutorily homeless people.* Mainly families, accepted by local authorities for rehousing and either placed directly into permanent housing association or local authority accommodation (at which point they cease to be homeless) or awaiting permanent accommodation in temporary housing (still viewed as homeless). This group also includes 'vulnerable' households and individuals.
2 *Single homeless people.* Mainly single men, although more young people and more women are joining this group, who have either been refused or have not sought assistance under the 1985 Act and are living in hostels or similar provision. Members of this group relatively often have poor health status and other 'vulnerable' characteristics.
3 *People sleeping rough.* Again, mainly single men, although the numbers of young people and women are rising in this group as well. Characterised by very poor health status, this minority of homeless people represents the worst extreme of homelessness.

Hidden homelessness

While the main focus of the debate and the basis of currently used definitions of homelessness in the United Kingdom is around the homelessness legislation, there are also definitional issues around the nature of homelessness itself. These issues do not arise while arguing about or discussing which homeless people should receive assistance; rather, they arise in the discussion of the nature of homelessness itself.

The definition of homelessness given in the 1977 Act and subsequently in the 1985 Act is as follows:

> someone is homeless if there is no accommodation in England, Wales or Scotland which that person can reasonably occupy together with anyone else who normally lives with them as a member of their family or in circumstances in which it is reasonable for that person to do so
>
> (Department of the Environment 1991)

This definition will be superseded with the new version contained in Section 175 of the 1996 Housing Act. This new version makes a number of changes, such as stating that the person must have no accommodation 'in the United Kingdom or elsewhere' that they can reasonably occupy, but is essentially the same.

Issues arise around how accommodation that someone can 'reasonably occupy' is defined. Essentially, these arguments are about the extent to which overcrowding or insecurity of tenure are defined as 'poor housing conditions' or as 'homelessness'. Some argue that overcrowding, if severe enough (sleeping on someone's floor, a younger couple living in one partner's parental home and so on), is a form of homelessness. The homelessness legislation allows for people who are threatened with homelessness, and a person or a household can be accommodated on that basis, before they become actually homeless. It does not, however, explicitly allow for overcrowding, except in the general sense of whether or not accommodation is somewhere in which an applicant can reasonably be expected to live, with local authorities interpreting what is 'reasonable'. Naturally, demonstrating imminent homelessness or unacceptable overcrowding is not enough in itself and a homeless person or household seeking assistance must still be in priority need, demonstrate a local connection and so forth.

'Hidden' homelessness is usually defined as people who are living in insecure accommodation and who are regarded as either a concealed or as a potential household. Concealed households are those that share accommodation with at least one other household. Potential households are those in which a concealed household or a member or members of an existing household wish to live separately.

There are a number of problems with the concept of hidden homelessness. The most fundamental one is that no one is exactly sure what it means, since seemingly almost *any* form of housing need, such as a teenager wanting a place of their own, can fall within its definitions. There is a danger that by referring to all housing need as a form of homelessness, the unique nature and distress of actual homelessness becomes lost. Overcrowding, poor housing conditions and insecurity of tenure are all very important problems affecting hundreds of thousands, if not millions, of people, but apart from their most extreme manifestations, they cannot be regarded as homelessness. Quite simply, being poorly housed is one thing, having nowhere at all to live is something else. What is referred to as hidden homelessness is generally not homelessness at all, but instead encompasses moderate to severe housing need, something that falls outside the scope of the present volume (although see the discussion in Ford, this volume).

MEASURING HOMELESSNESS

The lack of consensus about what exactly constitutes homelessness, the distinction made between non-statutory homelessness and statutory homelessness and the logistical difficulties of measurement combine in creating a situation in which data on homelessness that could be regarded as comprehensive and reliable do not currently exist. What follows then is an attempt to piece together the data which do exist but with due recognition of the multitude of caveats that such an undertaking involves.

People sleeping rough

The information on the number of people sleeping rough ranges from poor to non-existent. This is mainly because people sleeping rough are very difficult to count and because no agency with sufficient resources has ever tried to do it. People sleeping rough tend to be mobile (Vincent *et al.* 1993, 1995) and they also spend periods on and off the street, some making use of night shelters and other accommodation when they can get access to it. More vulnerable sections of the population sleeping rough, such as people from ethnic minorities and women, may not be revealed to their full extent because they do not use the provision for people sleeping rough such as winter or night shelters which tend to be full of white males (CRASH 1995, 1996; Davies *et al.* 1996).

Walking around cities at night with a clipboard, the usual method employed to count the population within an area who are sleeping rough, is inherently unreliable. This is mainly because the 'methodology' employed, an imprecise snapshot over one or two nights, cannot hope to represent the actual numbers of people sleeping rough (if nothing else because the population is known to fluctuate). In addition, some of the counts are carried out by organisations without research skills that are seeking to make a political point about the level of homelessness or raise money, producing figures that have to be treated with great caution. There have been attempts to bring more methodological rigour into counting street homeless populations, such as the attempt by Fisher *et al.* (1994) to employ the 'capture, recapture' methods used for estimating numbers of animals in the wild, although employing such techniques might be thought to dehumanise homeless people. The counts employed by the 1991 Census have been acknowledged by OPCS (1991) as an underestimate because they were little more (and sometimes less) than street counts.

The number of people experiencing rough sleeping during a given year probably reaches well into the thousands. The number of people experiencing rough sleeping on any given night is certainly a lot less, probably in the low thousands, maybe even under a thousand, but there are no real data to give a clear idea. Certainly, street homelessness is present in the United Kingdom in a way that has not been seen since before the Second World War, and anyone living in London only has to visit the Bull Ring or parts of the West End to see it. The same applies in every other major city. Intervention by government on a considerable scale, through the Homeless Mentally Ill Initiative and the Rough Sleepers Initiative (RSI), phases one and two, have also not solved the problem within London (Randall and Brown 1993). The scale of the problem is perhaps best illustrated by a government that is generally reluctant about public spending on welfare provision continuing to direct resources at the problem with RSI III, which will include expenditure outside London and put total expenditure on rough sleeping close to the £200 million mark.

Information on the lifestyles, health status and characteristics of people who spend some or most of their time sleeping rough is generally quite good. The findings of Anderson *et al.* (1993) which are described by Kemp and Bines within this volume and the detailed qualitative studies carried out by Vincent, Deacon and others of single homeless men (Dant and Deacon 1989; Vincent *et al.* 1993, 1995) are the reason why the estimates of the numbers of people sleeping rough are treated with caution. It is known that homeless people spend periods on and off the street and that they are often highly mobile.

Single homeless people

Single homeless people who are not sleeping rough are a diverse population and this creates the first problem in measurement. It has been argued above that the term 'hidden homelessness' is a misnomer, because the interpretation of 'homelessness' it employs is so wide as to encompass all forms of housing need. However, single homelessness will probably always be something that has fuzzy definitional edges, and deciding where the line between homelessness and extreme housing need is located will never be straightforward. Other than restating the argument that homelessness means having no home that one can reasonably live in, and that it does not encompass other forms of housing need, this volume cannot provide an answer to what is ultimately an ideological debate about when people in housing need should be assisted.

However, even if one dodges around the really difficult question of where to draw the line by stating that single homeless people are individuals *without accommodation that they can reasonably occupy*, measurement is still difficult. When individuals are staying within accommodation designed for homeless people or short stays, it is simple to define them as homeless. Anyone living in a hostel, bed and breakfast accommodation (B&B), a women's refuge, a direct access hostel or night shelter can be regarded as being among the single homeless population. Yet when they are living in a form of housing, their numbers and needs become very difficult to determine because there are very limited data and because agreement about where homelessness begins and ends has not yet been arrived at.

Again, a central problem in measurement is that the single homeless population is in a state of flux. Some people experience homelessness for years, sometimes even decades (Vincent *et al.* 1995), but many experience it periodically or enter the homeless population for a period and then leave it (Anderson *et al.* 1993). Indeed, Burrows (this volume) shows that some 4.3 per cent of all current heads of household in England have experienced (self-defined) periods of homelessness at some time in the last decade. Measurement, as with the population of people sleeping rough, is difficult because the target is constantly moving and changing shape.

It is possible to speculate about what the numbers of single home-less people may be: a recent estimate of total homelessness in Lon-don (Pleace and Quilgars 1996) put the total number of homeless people at around 106,000 in the last quarter of 1995. Within this fig-ure there were 15,000 people living in hostels and 11,000 living in squats. It is possible to surmise that most of these people were sin-gle, giving a total of (very approximately) 26,000 single homeless people in London alone.

This figure is certainly an underestimate, because the data avail-able were limited and it could be raised or lowered by including or excluding another 3,600 people using winter shelters, direct access hostels or night shelters, most of whom were probably spending at least some of their time sleeping rough – CRASH monitoring of the winter shelters in London found that only 18 per cent of women and 8 per cent of men using them had never slept rough – 11 per cent overall (CRASH 1996). It is also a figure covering only one point in time; the number of single homeless people in London over the course of a year will be much higher because people are constantly entering and leaving the single homeless population.

Extrapolating from this very rough estimate for London is not really possible because the data available are too limited, but even given that London has higher levels of homelessness than other areas in the United Kingdom, the numbers experiencing single non-statutory homelessness at any one time can probably be counted in the tens of thousands.

Statutory homelessness

It is perhaps with some sense of relief that the discussion can move on to the levels of statutory homelessness in England. At the time of writing, every local authority fills in quite lengthy returns, called the P1E, every quarter, supplying details of the homeless households it has accepted and rehoused under the 1985 Housing Act. Rather than guesswork that verges on being simply speculative, there are exten-sive data to draw upon on statutory homelessness, which do almost certainly account for the bulk of homelessness in England. Burrows (this volume), for example, shows that of the 4.3 per cent of current heads of household in England who had perceived themselves to be homeless in the last ten years almost 77 per cent had approached a local authority as homeless and of these just over 76 per cent were accepted as statutorily homeless.

Data on statutory homelessness collected for the P1E returns do still need to be treated with caution because they are collected on *households* rather than on *individuals*. A two- or three-person household is recorded as one 'acceptance' under the Act, with little information being collected on that household (even to the extent that one cannot find out how many people are in it, how old they are, what gender they are or what their ethnic origin is). A single homeless person accepted as statutorily homeless is recorded in the same way, as a single acceptance. The Department of the Environment (DoE) figures thus report levels of homelessness acceptances well under 200,000 households; however, in the last year for which data on household size were available (in 1992, from another statistical source) the 143,000 acceptances were found actually to represent more than 400,000 people (Standing Conference on Public Health 1994: 18).

The number of acceptances under the homelessness legislation rose dramatically after the first of the succession of Conservative governments came to power in 1979. At the time, this was widely associated with two policies. First, the decision to introduce the Right to Buy for council tenants at a national level, which effectively removed much of the better social housing stock in the United Kingdom over a period of a few years. Second, local authority subsidy was first cut and then removed, with all new social housing development shifting to the much smaller housing association sector. As Table 1.1 shows, since 1991 the figures have recently been falling (from 144,780 in 1991 to 120,810 in 1995, but still more than double the 1979 level), and the government has claimed that this is a result of its housing policies. Critics have argued that local authority and housing association stock is now so limited that authorities are being forced to interpret the homelessness legislation in an increasingly restrictive way (Butler *et al.* 1994).

The regional distribution of statutory acceptances shows that the apparent national decline in levels is not uniform. Table 1.2 shows the distribution of homelessness acceptances under the 1985 Housing Act across the main regions of England over the period 1991–95. The fall in the North West is the highest, with almost a third fewer acceptances in 1995 compared with 1991 and large falls are also apparent in the North East and London (although Greater London still accounted for 22 per cent of all acceptances in 1995 by itself and has a much higher level of acceptances per 1,000 households than the rest of England, 9.8 compared to 6.2 in 1994 (Pleace and Quilgars 1996: 16)). In one area, the South West, the number of acceptances

Table 1.1 Households accepted as statutorily homeless, England,
        1984–95

Year	No. of acceptances	% change on previous year
1984	80,500	+6.7
1985	91,010	+13.1
1986	100,490	+10.4
1987	109,170	+8.6
1988	113,770	+4.2
1989	122,180	+7.4
1990	140,350	+14.9
1991	144,780	+3.2
1992	142,890	−1.3
1993	132,380	−7.4
1994	122,460	−7.5
1995	120,810	−1.3

Source: Department of the Environment (1996) *Information Bulletin*, London:
Government Statistical Service. Own analysis

rose over the same period – see also Burrows (this volume) – and in
the Eastern, West Midlands and South Eastern regions there has been
little variation. Again, the extent to which the changes in the North
and London are the function of a decline in actual homelessness or
the result of increasingly strict definition of statutory homelessness
by authorities with increasingly limited stock of their own, and
declining access to housing association property, is the subject of
much debate and argument.

By examining the raw data sent into the Department of the Environment for the 1995 P1E returns it is also possible to look at the distribution of statutory homelessness across different types of local
authority. Urban authorities accept higher numbers of statutorily
homeless households than district councils. In 1995, according to the
raw data sent to the DoE, 66 metropolitan districts and London boroughs
accepted 51 per cent of all the homeless households accommodated
under the 1985 Housing Act, compared with the 49 per cent accepted
by 293 city and district councils. Some have interpreted this pattern of
a higher level of urban acceptances as a function of political control,
with more enlightened urban authorities being more liberal in their
acceptance criteria than authorities in rural and semi-rural areas. This
argument may well explain some amount of variation, but it is also
likely that the greater availability of stock within urban areas allows
authorities to accept proportionately more homeless households.

Table 1.2 Regional distribution of statutory homelessness, 1991–95

Region	1991	1992	1993	1994	1995	% change 1991–95
North East	8,450	7,710	7,080	6,260	6,300	−25.44
Yorks & Humber	13,080	14,820	13,650	11,330	10,210	−21.94
East Midlands	10,300	10,770	10,370	9,070	9,040	−12.23
Eastern	8,830	9,420	9,080	8,580	8,800	−0.34
London	37,060	37,840	31,890	28,920	26,610	−28.20
South East	14,410	13,360	13,140	13,540	14,250	−1.11
South West	9,330	9,100	9,470	9,300	10,050	+7.72
West Midlands	18,400	17,520	17,060	16,430	18,090	−1.68
North West	21,330	18,730	17,040	15,600	14,480	−32.11
Merseyside	3,590	3,620	3,600	3,430	2,980	−16.99
England	144,780	142,890	132,380	122,460	120,810	−16.56

Source: Department of the Environment (1996) *Information Bulletin*, London: Government Statistical Service. Own analysis

This pattern of acceptances becomes particularly interesting when the characteristics of the households which are accepted under the homelessness legislation are examined. Table 1.3 shows the broad characteristics of the households accepted in 1995 and also includes estimates from the raw P1E data for that year showing the average acceptances of these household types in different kinds of authorities. The higher overall acceptances made by large urban authorities were reflected in much higher acceptance levels of vulnerable households. This can be further illustrated by examining the levels of acceptance in terms of households that were primarily accepted as in priority need because they contained children. Across England as a whole in 1995, approximately 74 per cent of acceptances were households containing children and 24 per cent were 'vulnerable' households, which are mainly lone homeless people. In the district and smaller city councils, the figures were close to this national level (75 per cent and 23 per cent), but in Outer London more vulnerable households were accepted (31 per cent) and in the Metropolitan Districts the figure rose to 33 per cent, while in Inner London it was 38 per cent. Statutory single homelessness is therefore concentrated in urban areas, especially within Inner London, which has especially high levels of acceptance of people with mental health problems compared with other areas.

Table 1.3 Characteristics of statutorily homeless households and average estimated acceptances by local authority type, 1995

Reason for priority need	No.	District and city councils[1] average	Metropolitan districts average	Outer London average	Inner London average	England average
Dependent children	67,100	116	469	331	450	173
Member pregnant	13,350	22	82	85	142	34
Vulnerable older person	5,950	11	32	30	54	15
Disabled person	6,470	9	33	56	96	17
Mental health problem or learning difficulty	7,250	9	47	56	101	19
Vulnerable young person	3,620	4	47	9	21	9
Person(s) escaping domestic violence	7,650	7	140	14	30	22
Other special reason[2]	4,210	4	99	19	32	15

Sources: Department of the Environment (1995) Households Found Accommodation Under the Homelessness Legislation: England and Department of the Environment, P1E (Homelessness) Returns for 1995. Own analysis (excludes non-responding authorities)

Notes:
1 Includes new unitary authorities
2 People accepted because of serious and/or debilitating illness, such as HIV. Some authorities accepted vulnerable categories of ex-offender and other vulnerable groups under the code of guidance to the 1985 Housing Act

THE STRUCTURE OF THE VOLUME

Many of the themes and issues discussed in this introductory chapter are elaborated upon elsewhere in the volume. The chapters by Lowe (Chapter 2) and Neale (Chapter 3) develop in some detail the legal and definitional issues surrounding homelessness and link these debates to contemporary theorisations of the phenomena.

The chapters by Burrows (Chapter 4) and Kemp (Chapter 5) provide some additional statistical material to the aggregate data provided in this chapter by examining survey data on the experience of homelessness in the population as a whole and the characteristics of single homeless people in England.

The chapter by Ford (Chapter 6) examines the relationship between the unsustainability of owner occupation and homelessness, and in so doing focuses upon the needs of homeless families. The chapter by Higate (Chapter 7), by contrast, is more conceptual and introduces some provocative ideas about the plight of homelessness amongst one particular group – ex-servicemen – who have received much publicity in recent years (Randall and Brown 1994). Carlisle (Chapter 8) examines another specific group – ex-prisoners – who, although they have not received so much publicity, face huge problems securing adequate accommodation.

The chapters by Bines (Chapter 9) and Pleace and Quilgars (Chapter 10) both examine the relationship between homelessness and health. The chapter by Bines is a summary of her widely cited work on the impact of homelessness on health status, whilst the chapter by Pleace and Quilgars concentrates on issues of access to health care.

The next five chapters all examine in some detail particular policy responses to various aspects of homelessness. Pleace (Chapter 11) examines policies aimed at rehousing single homeless people. Rugg (Chapter 12) offers an evaluation of policies designed to assist homeless people gain access to accommodation in the private rented sector (PRS), whilst Bevan and Rhodes (Chapter 13) examine the capacity of the PRS to house homeless households. Neale (Chapter 14) evaluates the role played by hostels in alleviating homelessness, whilst Quilgars and Anderson (Chapter 15) evaluate a more recent and innovative response – that of foyers.

The volume concludes with a chapter by Oldman (Chapter 16) which considers contemporary policies towards homelessness in a slightly wider context. In particular, the chapter considers some of the positive and negative aspects of the necessity for agencies to work together jointly when implementing policies aimed at helping homeless people.

CONCLUDING COMMENTS

The problem of homelessness is deeply emblematic of the sort of society that we now live in. What other social phenomena better epitomises the end of the modernist project than the premodern conditions of existence experienced by so many people who are homeless? Surely it is only under conditions of postmodernity that the obscene juxtaposition of street homelessness alongside hyper-dynamic technological developments could occur within such close proximity? Surely it is only under conditions of postmodernity that societies able to produce the sort of scientific and technological developments we now witness on an almost daily basis are, at the same time, seemingly unable to provide for the most basic needs – shelter, warmth, food – of substantial numbers of 'citizens' (Davis 1992; Lash and Urry 1994; Burrows 1997)? Is not the policy response to homelessness also indicative of the postmodern thesis that contemporary discourses are exhausted? It is not only post-modern cultural artefacts (architecture, music, art, novels, cinema and so on) which now so often appear as tired rehashes of older, originally more vibrant, elements. The same also appears to be the case in the fields of politics and social policy (Gibbins 1989). Somehow we now seem powerless at the level of social policy to address basic human needs. It is as if we have become so embroiled in the complexities of social and cultural life, and so dominated by individualistic discourses, that the recognition of real need has become obscured (Carter 1997). Surely it can only be under post-modern conditions that policy interventions based upon providing more affordable and decent housing could have become almost unthinkable?

As will be apparent to the reader, this is a volume largely rooted in a tradition of empirical social policy research rather than the complexities of debates about the postmodern condition. As such it provides a largely dispassionate consideration of various aspects of homelessness in contemporary Britain. However, having stated that, it is hoped that it will provide both conceptual and empirical materials which will be of use to all those people who are still unfashionable enough to want to change things for the better.

NOTES

1 The CHP was formed in 1990 under the Directorship of Professor Peter Kemp in order to focus in one place research on housing and social policy within the University of York. The work of the Centre currently focuses on five main themes: the management and funding of rented housing; the changing nature and sustainability of owner occupation; housing aspects of community care and health; affordability and the relationship between housing and social security; and, the theme of this volume, homelessness and access to housing. Researchers in the Centre currently come from backgrounds in social policy, sociology, political science and history. Throughout its history the work of the Centre has aimed to produce high-quality housing policy research funded by the Department of the Environment, the Department of Social Security, the Joseph Rowntree Foundation, the King's Fund, the Housing Corporation, the Rural Development Commission and a plethora of other organisations. Further details about the work of the CHP can be obtained by writing to the Administrator, Centre for Housing Policy, University of York, Heslington, York, YO1 5DD, or via the World Wide Web – http://www.york.ac.uk/inst/chp/.
2 This volume was prepared in late 1996.

Chapter 2

Homelessness and the law

Stuart Lowe

Homelessness is one of those areas of social policy in which law and policy operate cheek by jowl, and it is the purpose of this chapter to show the nature and consequences of this interaction.[1] Writing in the autumn of 1996 is a particularly poignant moment for such an assessment because the Housing Act 1996, which reached the statute books in June, provides *inter alia* for dramatic changes to the legal duties of local authorities established in the Housing (Homeless Person) Act 1977. Under the 1977 system local housing authorities for the first time acquired duties to provide permanent accommodation for a variety of people in need. Section VII of the Housing Act 1996 (operative from 1 January 1997) to all intents and purposes abolishes these duties with homeless families being offered only temporary assistance and this under only very strictly defined circumstances. The two decades from 1977 to 1997 would thus seem to form a distinct historical phase and one aim of the chapter is to describe and comment on the legal aspects of the new system and how it differs from the old.

A second aim of the chapter is to describe the strong and long-run continuities in the treatment of homeless and destitute people. They have normally been excluded and marginalised from mainstream society, and since the advent of the Victorian Poor Law a specialised conceptual framework and language has evolved and become embedded in English social thought. The homeless are spoken of in terms of their 'eligibility' for help, whether they are 'deserving' or 'undeserving', whether they have 'local connections', and a punitive aspect is fearfully present in the concept 'less eligibility'. When it came to the abolition of the Poor Law in 1948 this vocabulary of social exclusion and marginalisation was carried forward into the legislative framework. Indeed, these and other related concepts have been minutely scrutinised in case law that developed around the basic

statutes. The law itself is not culpable, however, but has been a civil-
ising influence with a role to clarify, correct errors, control malad-
ministration and the introduction of irrelevancies and prejudices.
Through this process law has sought to develop a consistent and
nationally cohesive system in a situation fraught with local variations
in practice.

Read in this long view, Part VII of the Housing Act 1996 is much
more in tune with the miserly and punitive spirit of the Poor Law
than the current system, and the conceptual and legal framework of
this new legislation is very much a throwback to the position as it
was at the time of the National Assistance Act 1948 which gave local
authorities duties to house only actually roofless people. The language of social exclusion resonates through both statutes and was
never far below the surface of the 1977 system despite its relatively
progressive stance.

The first section of the chapter explores the Poor Law legacy. The
second section outlines the legal and policy context leading up to the
implementation of the National Assistance Act 1948, then to the
1977 system. The final part of the chapter outlines briefly the main
developments to the current system arising from the Housing Act
1996, followed by a concluding commentary about the implications
of the new statute.

THE POOR LAW HERITAGE

The Poor Law system, as it was administered in England, began in
1563, when parishes were allowed to impose a tax to cater for the
needs of its destitute and homeless families. In essence this was a
charitable approach (although not in any sense implying generosity)
overseen by JPs and church vestry officials – a system with its roots
very much in the centuries-old feudal tradition with obligations and
duties owed to each and all at every level of society. Aid came in the
form either of domiciliary support, commonly known as 'outdoor
relief', or through special provision in residential houses in which
the aged and infirm could be gathered and the able-bodied given support while they sought work. It was not until 1722 that parishes were
allowed to open 'workhouses' for the more generally destitute, often
through the use of private contractors (see National Assistance Act
1948; Glastonbury 1971).

The Law of Settlement and Removal 1662 allowed parishes to
exclude from parish relief anyone who could not prove a local con-

nection or some right of settlement. The system was highly dependent, of course, on the benevolence of local landowners, although, as
Gauldie points out, they often adopted a role of 'niggardly dispensa-
tion' to small numbers of people than general charitableness to all
comers. Indeed, to avoid the potential burden of support for outdoor
relief it was common practice for landowners to demolish unused
cottages (Gauldie 1974: 34–45). The administration of outdoor relief
was always going to be a problem, simply because the fact of its provision was bound to encourage demand in an era when desperate and
life-threatening poverty was endemic. In this equation the demand
and supply cycle for labour and the general well-being of local
economies were also important factors. Then, as now, local practices
varied very considerably.

Parishes became much stricter in the application of the Vagrancy
Laws and Laws of Settlement as the population grew and became
increasingly mobile under the impact of the Agricultural and then the
Industrial Revolutions. In practice only the able-bodied unemployed
were eligible for relief notwithstanding the destitution of large parts
of the urban and rural *employed* population. Growing demands on the
system gradually gave rise to pressure for change, and accordingly a
Royal Commission was set up in 1832 to investigate what was to be
done. Many of its recommendations were incorporated into the Poor
Law Amendment Act 1834.

The 1834 Act is one of the great moments of English social policy.
It marks a fundamental turning point from a system of misguided and
half-hearted benevolence based essentially on the power of local
landowners and clergy, to a determination by the national state appa-
ratus to rid society of the moral scourge of poverty by its ruthless
subjugation. Its central purpose was to end outdoor relief and concentrate assistance through centrally organised workhouses. The condition of 'less eligibility' was designed to ensure that workhouse
occupants were 'in no case so eligible as the conditions of persons of
the lowest class subsisting on the fruits of their own industry'. Such
a state of life was destined to be deplorably poor and degrading
because rural and urban wages were already intolerably low; indeed,
as Chadwick, the first secretary to the new Poor Law Commission,
acknowledged, 'The diet of the workhouse almost always exceeds
that of the cottage' (quoted in Finer 1952: 83). In order to create
the necessary deterrence other strictly worked-out rules were
imposed; workhouse clothes were compulsory, meals were eaten in
silence, funeral bells were not rung for the workhouse dead, whose

final resting place was in unmarked paupers' graves. The dread with which working-class families came to view the workhouse was compounded by a system of 'classification'. The intention was to weed out the inept and ignorant poor from those more able to stand on their own two feet. Such separation was in practice not easily administered. Far easier was to segregate people by age and sex. Children were taken from their mothers, husbands and wives were separated and families broken up.

This is not the place to debate further the operation of the Poor Law. Suffice it to say that its existence had a devastating effect on the lives of generations and millions of poor working-class families. As one measure of the scale of things Townsend pointed to the fact that as late as 1911 a quarter of all single men over the age of 65 lived in casual wards of workhouse infirmaries (Townsend 1964). Following the precept of 'classification', the separation of elderly sick and frail men and women was very typical of the times. It figured prominently in the social reforms of the Liberal governments and generally through the inter-war period, although under the guise of the 'break-up' of the Poor Law. At this time it was held that destitution was a product not of family life *per se* but of the failure of some aspect of the education, pensions, health or manpower policies and it followed that specialised, targeted services needed to be devised to overcome such problems. This approach was meant to prefigure the end of the Poor Law system; however, it merely signalled the long-term demise of the workhouse not its immediate end. As Townsend observed,

> between 1910 and 1946 . . . the population aged 65 and over more than doubled and by 1946 the number of old people who were living in former workhouses, now run as public assistance institutions or as general or chronic sick hospitals, was greater than what it was at the turn of the century.
>
> (Townsend 1964: 17)

Indeed, it was not until the National Assistance Act 1948 that the Poor Law was abolished, and even then only in name, for many of the practices of social exclusion, stigmatisation and outright punishment were less easily confined to the dustbins of history, none more so than in the treatment of homeless families.

The National Assistance Act was not in practice a solution to the needs of homeless families because it continued much of the muddled thinking about the nature of homelessness and did not create a comprehensive, national framework for dealing with the problem.

Indeed, the statutory provision was designed only to deal with homeless families in the most narrow sense of being actually 'roofless', and then effectively only as a result of acute emergencies. Homelessness arising from a simple lack of available housing did not fall within the law's purview – see below the case of *Southwark LBC* v. *Williams*. The plight of the homeless was forgotten and subsumed in the desperate shortage of housing that followed the conclusion of the war. The post-war shortage of dwellings was estimated at something over 2 million, and the next two decades were spent in a political 'numbers game' trying to reduce this huge back-log.

Section 2 (1) of the Act created the National Assistance Board with duties to provide reception centres for the unsettled. The wandering homeless were thus provided for through the new national body while other forms of homelessness fell to the responsibility of local authority welfare departments. Local *housing* authorities had no duties in relation to the homeless. Section 21 (1) (b) created a duty (since repealed) to provide 'temporary accommodation for persons who are in urgent need thereof, being need arising in circumstances which could not reasonably have been foreseen . . .'. There were several difficulties with the Section 21 duties. First of all, temporary accommodation was not provided for in local authority budgets and they were left with little more than old war-time buildings – nissen huts and other ex-Forces accommodation – for the fulfilment of these responsibilities. Second, the legal nature of the responsibilities was not clearly defined. For example, there was no explanation or guidance about what precisely was 'urgent need' or 'unforeseen circumstances', and by the 1970s the courts had determined that there was no *enforceable* duty on local authorities (see *Southwark LBC* v. *Williams* [1971] Ch 734). Third, and largely as a result of those two factors, there continued in practice to be a great deal of variation between local authorities, and within authorities the administrative and legal void between housing and welfare departments was intensified.

As there was very little else to fall back on, the tried and tested processes for dealing with the homeless continued unabated. Aneurin Bevan's assertion that 'The workhouse is doomed' was very far from the reality. Families were broken up, ex-servicemen were recruited to be hostel wardens and the principle of less eligibility ensured that life in 'temporary accommodation' was bleak and demeaning. As Glastonbury points out, a fundamental problem was that there was still no agreement about the nature of the homelessness problem, with central government determined, against all evidence, to interpret 'unforeseen circumstances' in the most literal way possible – usually meaning 'fire and flood' (Glastonbury 1971).

Despite the attempt by government to define the problem out of existence the number of people living in temporary accommodation began to rise dramatically in the 1960s. Greve showed that the number of homeless families in Inner London rose by 51 per cent between 1966 and 1970, and Glastonbury found evidence of a 300 per cent increase in a sample of local authorities in South Wales and the south-west of England (Greve *et al.* 1971; Glastonbury 1971). Moreover, the screening in 1966 of the famous documentary drama *Cathy Come Home* about a homeless single parent and, subsequently, the setting up of the pressure group Shelter, created a much higher profile for the issue. Under pressure from public opinion and fuelled by the findings of the research community the system began to crack. In the early 1970s the situation reached new depths of absurdity.

Under Section 195 of the Local Government Act 1972 the duty under Section 21 (1) of the National Assistance Act was converted to a discretion (in line with the case law). This, of course, was no solution because the problem did not simply go away. In 1974 a joint DHSS and DoE Circular (No. 18/74) entitled 'Homelessness' stated that 'provision of suitable accommodation for the homeless in future be undertaken . . . by housing authorities'. But shortly afterwards the Secretary of State for Social Services issued a local authority circular (No13/74) *re-imposing* the duty to provide temporary accommodation on social services departments. The situation was little short of farcical. It was obvious that changes to the law were urgently needed, and it was through the medium of a Private Member's Bill – that of the Liberal MP Stephen Ross, based on a Department of the Environment draft – that the foundations of the Housing (Homeless Persons) Act 1977 was based. Although enjoying all-party support, the Bill was heavily amended in its passage through Parliament due largely to the fears of a number of Conservative MPs and some local authorities of queue jumping, with families moving themselves round the country in pursuit of accommodation through this new system of provision, the same argument that re-appeared in the 1990s to justify the abolition of the core of the 1977 system in the Housing Act 1996.

THE 1977–97 SYSTEM

The 1977 Act recognised for the first time that homelessness was a *housing* problem, and homeless families – albeit of narrowly defined categories – were given statutory rights to permanent, secure accommodation provided by local authorities. Many of the attitudes and practices inherited from the past were not so easily eradicated. A complex case law developed around the Housing (Homeless Persons) Act, in which every nuance of language and turn of phrase has been tested and re-tested, and even the basic duty of provision persistently (and ultimately successfully) challenged by some local authorities. The law tried to develop a consistency of behaviour and interpretation across the country, as the extension of citizenship rights to homeless families surely implied, and thus to reverse the age-old tradition of local discretions. The DoE published a Code of Guidance which, while not itself 'law', tried to impose a degree of common practice. The Code also became the subject of much litigation and has been rewritten three times since it was first published, a third edition (DoE 1991) being much more detailed than its predecessors in order to 'tighten up' implementation procedures.

The 1977 Act was codified with the rest of the housing legislation in 1985 and became Part III of the Housing Act 1985. It was amended soon afterwards by the Housing and Planning Act 1986. In 1989 the government published a review of the legislation and decided to maintain the existing law with some management changes and improvements in inter-agency co-operation. It was recognised that the Code of Guidance needed strengthening to ensure a more even-handed approach by the authorities, and the new third edition was published in 1991. New duties to homeless people were also developed through the Children Act 1989 and the NHS and Community Care Act 1990, empowering and sometimes requiring social services departments to provide accommodation for 18-year-olds (and older 'children' if necessary) who are in need of care. The Secretary of State was also required to provide and maintain resettlement units. Thus by the mid-1990s new layers of jurisdiction were once again in operation with a danger of the recurrence of the pre-1977 situation when people would be shuttled between departments.

Essentially the 1985 system established a series of hurdles over which applicants had to jump successfully before the authority owed them a duty to provide permanent secure accommodation. These are described in detail elsewhere (Hughes and Lowe, 1995: chap. 5), and very useful contextual material is to be found in Clapham *et al.* (1990). The aim here is simply to sketch the main elements of the system because, although Part VII of the Housing Act 1996 repeals Part III of the 1985 Act, many provisions are re-enacted in the new legislation albeit with changes and a number of radical modifications (and some additions).

The first hurdle to be crossed is the determination of whether or not the applicant is actually a homeless person. This is defined in Section 58, and the new edition of the Code of Guidance (DoE 1991) gives further detail with a list of criteria – for example, when a woman is at risk of serious assault, the physical conditions of the current accommodation and/or overcrowding are not 'reasonable' and this includes people threatened with homelessness within twenty-eight days. Such people may be under threat of eviction through a court order, not able to gain access to the accommodation and other similar situations. Clearly, the precise circumstances must be taken into account and this is generally the position followed by the law. For example, a pregnant woman following medical advice that her tenancy of a beach hut was not suitable joined a squat and was incorrectly refused accommodation by her local authority. The authority considered that she had 'accommodation' *(R.* v. *Median Borough Council, ex parte* Dee [1992]).

The Code of Guidance sets down the basis of procedure after initial contact has been made with timescales. The duty to accommodate depends on whether the applicant is in 'priority need' – defined as including pregnant women or people with whom she lives (for example, the father of the child); people with dependent children; people vulnerable due to old age, mental illness or some other disability; and people threatened with homelessness due to an emergency such as fire or flood. Priority need due to being vulnerable has been tested in the courts on many occasions and hangs on questions of degree and fact. For example, ex-offenders released from prison are not treated as vulnerable by some local authorities. Equally, there is no clear definition in relation to mentally ill people, and the case law turns in effect on whether or not a person is able to fend for themselves in circumstances in which a person of normal ability could cope without injury or harm.

Having jumped the hurdles of eligibility and priority need, the applicant then has to prove that they are not intentionally homeless. The wording of Section 60 also created a significant volume of judicial reviews. The test is whether or not a person 'deliberately does or fails to do anything in consequence of which he ceases to occupy accommodation which is available . . . and which it would have been reasonable for him to continue to occupy'. Typical of decisions here are whether someone affected by homelessness acquiesced in the situation. Mrs Spruce, for example, genuinely believed that her husband had paid off a rent arrears. When her husband was deemed intentionally homeless as a result of the arrears it was held that she was not party to this outcome. Local authority practice is variable on such issues and not inclined to generosity. In a recent study, 20 per cent of authorities considered that the termination of a short-term or holiday let was intentional. Rather curiously, only 16 per cent considered mortgage arrears as an intentional act but 49 per cent viewed rent arrears in this way (Butler *et al.* 1994).

After passing the test of eligibility, priority need and intentionality, it is generally held that the full duty of provision is due under the law. The authority may, however, make an inquiry about whether the person has a local connection with another authority and may, if so found, refer the person to this other authority provided there is no threat of domestic violence. According to the Local Authority Agreement (1979), a local connection implies being resident in an area for at least six out of the preceding twelve months, although this is a rule of practice rather than a requirement of the law.

If in the end the applicant is deemed not to be owed the duty of provision the authority has subsequent duties normally involving the provision of information and advice. Most authorities appear to comply with the Code of Guidance on this, but nearly 40 per cent of authorities do not offer arrears and debt advice (Butler *et al.* 1994). Authorities also have to provide *temporary* accommodation in two circumstances: pending the outcome of their inquiries, and if an applicant is in a priority-need category but found to be intentionally homeless.

THE 1997 SYSTEM

The government signalled its intention to change radically the duties contained in Part III of the Housing Act 1985 in a Consultation Paper issued in January 1994 , 'Access to local authority and housing association tenancies' (DoE 1994a). This paper, despite the almost overwhelming opposition to it (there were over 10,000 responses), formed the basis of the system.

Three clear lines of argument are made, although none of them are strongly supported by evidence. First was that in some areas of the country, particularly in London, virtually all new social tenancies were allocated to homeless households. In fact, during 1994–95 about 40 per cent of social tenancies allocated by local authorities went to homeless households. Nevertheless this is still a high figure but is caused not by an increase in the number of homeless acceptances – some 120,000 in that year and a figure that had been stable for several years and was falling after a period of rapid growth following the 1977 Act – but by the decline in availability of re-lets. This was due to the sale of council houses under the Right to Buy legislation and the collapse of the local authority building programme (Bramley 1993).

Second was that homelessness was, in the words of the Consultation Paper, a 'fast-track' route into permanent accommodation, 'an attractive way into subsidised housing for those wishing to be re-housed'. Government spokesmen clearly believed that female single parents were distorting the system by queue jumping, and the paper talks at several points about 'married couples' as the normal situation within which family life should be conducted. There appears, however, to be no evidence that young women were deliberately becoming pregnant to queue jump the waiting list. Indeed, the study by Butler *et al.* (1994), conducted before the publication of the Consultation Paper, found that nearly 60 per cent of statutorily homeless households were already registered on council-house waiting lists. This would seem to imply a deterioration of circumstances rather than a deliberate ploy to gatecrash the system.

Third, it was argued that many of those accepted as homeless were not actually without homes – because the duties under the legislation were to rehouse groups not only without housing but in danger of losing settled accommodation. The number of people actually roofless, so it was argued, was relatively low. The figure of 2,700 rough sleepers counted in the 1991 Census (OPCS 1991) was cited as evidence of this 'fact', although it is known that this assessment was seriously flawed and the figure for rough sleepers is much higher. A rather more serious point is that the DoE's own figures showed that a high proportion of homelessness acceptances were the result of family disputes, with the implication that these circumstances would now fall outside the terms of the narrow definition of homelessness proposed and leave such people imprisoned in potentially traumatic relationships.

Thus, whatever the merits of the arguments, the Consultation Paper aimed several swinging blows at the 1977 system. On the one hand it was argued that there was widespread abuse of the waiting-list system by people who used homelessness as a way of leap-frogging ordinary applicants. It followed that the existing system had encour-

aged certain types of people to exploit statutory protections unjusti-
fiably. Accordingly, the paper argued for a redefinition of local
authority duties as solely the provision of emergency accommodation. The duty would become one of helping only those unintentionally homeless with no accommodation of any sort. Moreover, that
duty would not commence until an assessment of circumstances had
been completed (although this extremely hard-line view was eventually dropped). The second proposal restricted authorities' duties to a
limited period during which the applicants had to find a solution to
their housing problem themselves, either through a housing association, the ordinary waiting list or in the private rented sector (PRS). No
specific time limit was put on this in the Consultation Paper but in the
White Paper (DoE 1995a) that followed the duty was fixed at one
year, although it was subsequently changed to two years in the Act.

No mention was made in the Queen's Speech of November 1994
of a legislative proposal to enact the new system and for a time it
appeared that the government was having second thoughts. This
turned out to be only a pause due to the volume of the government's
legislative programme – including the aborted proposal to privatise
the Post Office – and the development of their other housing plans,
including the establishment of 'Housing Companies' progressively to
take over the management of council housing. A White Paper, 'Our
future homes', was subsequently published in June 1995 (DoE
1995a) and in relation to the homelessness issue brought forward in
revised form most of the Consultation Paper proposals: 'The proposals aim to introduce greater fairness into the allocation of long-term
tenancies in local authority and housing association homes while
retaining a safety net for families and vulnerable people who become
homeless unintentionally.'

The severe restriction of the existing duties was given further
impetus by a judgment of the House of Lords in the case of *R*. v.
London Borough of Brent ex parte Awua [1995] 3 ALL ER 493 in
which it was held that Part III of the 1985 Act did *not* intend to give
local authorities a duty to provide permanent accommodation; the
duty was only to secure suitable accommodation and this could be
for as little as twenty-eight days. Buoyed up by this judgment,
which turned on allegations of queue jumping, government drafts-
men proceeded to write the homelessness proposals into its Housing Bill (published in early 1996), and by the end of June the new
legislation passed onto the statute books as Part VII of the Housing
Act 1996.

PART VII OF THE HOUSING ACT 1996

Part VII of the Housing Act 1996 repeals and replaces Part III of the
Housing Act 1985. Many of the 1985 provisions are re-enacted
although subject to considerable change. The detail of its implementation is subject to the accompanying Regulations and the new Code
of Guidance which are currently being written and were due for publication in December 1996, the new system becoming operative on
1 January 1997. The force of the changes in the law is readily apparent in the statute and the clear duty in future is to secure only temporary accommodation – potentially in effect for only one year (see
below) and for a maximum of two years with re-application and new
inquiries. The aim is that this accommodation will be found normally
in the privately rented sector and possibly in housing association
property or the authorities' own stock. This duty can recur after two
years but is subject to a review of entitlement, and the clear assumption is that the households will during that time have solved their
problems.

An important change in the application procedure incorporates an
inquiry stage, during which the authority has to satisfy itself that the
person is *eligible* for assistance. Thus it is not enough merely to be
homeless. The applicant must also be eligible. Those who are ineligible include people from abroad and not entitled to social security
payments and *anyone else* deemed ineligible by the Secretary of
State. Asylum seekers or their dependants are also not eligible if they
have *any* accommodation, however temporary, available in the
United Kingdom. This section (186) has, however, already been met
by a judicial challenge in a recent case, in which it was held that
social services departments continue to have a duty under Section 21
(1) (a) of the National Assistance Act 1948 to accommodate destitute
asylum seekers. (*R.* v. *Hammersmith and Fulham LBC ex parte* M;
R. v. *Westminster CC ex parte* A, and *R.* v. *Lambeth LBC ex parte* P
and *ex parte* X [1996] *The Times,* 10 October (QBD)). This arises
because that section of the 1948 Act has never been repealed and has
remained dormant while the new layers of statute have been added
and taken precedence. A significant coach and horses would thus
appear to have been driven through the eligibility rules even before
the new system has started.

The definition of those in priority need – pregnant women, families with children, those vulnerable by age or disability, and people
homeless due to an emergency – are listed in Section 189 as before,

with no changes. The test of intentionality is, however, considerably added to. The basic test remains (see above), but a person is also deemed intentionally homeless if no other 'good reason' can be shown why they are homeless. Such circumstances would appear to be riven with potential for legal challenge, for what exactly is 'good reason'? A person is also intentionally homeless if they fail to secure 'suitable alternative accommodation' when it is available in the area in circumstances when they might reasonably be expected to obtain it (that is, it is not too expensive). Moreover, if having been given advice they fail to secure local accommodation, it would seem that the local authority, at their discretion, owes them no duty.

The idea of 'other suitable accommodation' (Section 197) gives the authorities a major 'get-out' provision for their duties to homeless people. If the *authority* considers that such accommodation is available, then all other duties owed fall. The potential for legal challenge and variation in local practice would seem to be very great, as 'other suitable' incorporates issues of tenure, the state of the local housing market and so on, as well as the applicant's personal circumstances. It seems fairly clear that from 1 January 1997 an authority that decides that suitable accommodation is available in their area – for example, in the PRS – have a discretion not to accommodate, only to advise and help.

Once all the hurdles have been crossed the 'full duty' is owed to the applicant. This duty is to continue for a minimum period of two years, after which the authority has a discretion, subject to new inquiries, to continue to accommodate. Thus the duty is in essence a duty to accommodate temporarily within a minimum span of two years. Under various circumstances this duty can cease – for example, if the person becomes intentionally homeless from the accommodation or if they refuse to accept an offer by the authority via the normal allocation system (one refusal is enough for the duty to fall).

Finally, Part VII makes it clear that the aim is to deprive statutorily homeless households of immediate access to council housing. The mechanism for achieving this is to *specify* (Section 207) the types of accommodation which the authority is to use in the discharge of its duties. For long-term arrangements the duty to accommodate is defined as referring to either hostels (as defined in Section 622 of the 1985 Act) or specifically leased accommodation, presumably mostly to be found in the PRS. Thus homeless families are *excluded* from council housing – except in so far as they become eligible through the normal waiting list.

Thus the twenty-year-old duty of local authorities to provide permanent accommodation for homeless people was to end on 31 December 1996. To gain access to the limited temporary help now to be available, mainly through a let in the PRS, applicants have to surmount several new hurdles. Not only do they have to satisfy the authorities that they are homeless but must now also be *eligible* (although, as we have seen, this requirement is already subject to judicial review). They must fall into one of the existing priority-need categories and be unintentionally homeless, inserting the proviso that no other 'good reason' can be cited against them and, of course, must have a sufficient local connection. And finally there is now an additional question which local authorities may ask: 'Is there other suitable accommodation available in the area?'

THE NEW SYSTEM IN PRACTICE

Bearing in mind that if an applicant fails to access such suitable alternative accommodation or refuses it, and given the prospect of life in hostels or short lets in the PRS, the future for homeless families after 1 January 1997 would appear to be bleak.

The proposals depend a great deal on suitable accommodation in the PRS being available. As the White Paper stated, 'A healthy private rented sector makes an important contribution to meeting the demand for housing. Local authorities have a strategic enabling role in supporting both landlords and tenants' (DoE 1995a). Thus a great deal of faith is being put in the ability of the PRS to mop up homeless people. Where otherwise do they go? There must, however, be considerable doubt whether this sector is able to perform such a role. It is beyond the brief of the chapter to examine this in detail but a few pointers should suffice. First, of course, it follows from the 'suitable accommodation' issue that such lets will be at market rents supported by housing benefit. This would, however, appear to be at variance with changes to the housing benefit system which became operative in January 1996. In particular, Statutory Instrument 1644 (DSS 1995) repeals the whole of Regulation 11 (of the Housing Benefit and Community Charge Regulations). Local authorities do not have to show that cheaper alternative accommodation is available before restricting housing benefit levels in their area. This would seem to cut completely across the ability of homeless households to access 'suitable available accommodation'. Moreover, under these changes prospective tenants may apply for a pre-tenancy determination of rent which uses the local authority rent officers to settle rent levels between tenant and landlord – an agreement that is binding for twelve months.

While in theory the aim of these measures is to exert downward pressure on rents in the private sector, it is by no means clear that this is happening. The key point here is that both these changes seem likely to *deter* landlords from entering tenancy agreements with households dependent on housing benefit. A recent study of landlords' behaviour concluded that many landlords considered 'letting accommodation to recipients [of housing benefit] a risky business which many . . . would prefer to be without' (Bevan *et al.* 1995). The likelihood of 'suitable alternative accommodation' being available through the PRS would thus seem to be reduced due to the government's own housing benefit policy. Further evidence of difficulties in the supply of accommodation in the PRS is contained in the study by Bevan and Rhodes which shows that those people registered as statutorily homeless in 1994 would have absorbed 25 per cent of all the lettings in the sector during that year, and in areas with a high proportion of council housing this figure was 60 per cent (Bevan and Rhodes 1997; this volume). There must be considerable question marks over the capability of the PRS to supply an adequate flow of accommodation for homeless households. The study reiterates the finding from their previous work that private landlords prefer not to let to tenants receiving housing benefit.

The White Paper urged local authorities to take a proactive role in developing links with private landlords. 'The more forward looking housing authorities are developing effective links with private sector landlords' (DoE 1995a). Derby Council was cited as an example of best practice through the creation of their voluntary register, and Colchester was praised for its rent deposit and guarantee schemes (covering losses caused by tenants and guaranteeing rent payments for a certain period). But the research by Butler *et al.* in 1993 showed that only 42 per cent of the local authorities in their study operated a lodgings register, 26 per cent had a rent deposit scheme and 11 per cent a rent guarantee scheme (Butler *et al.* 1994).

If, as we have seen, 60 per cent of homeless households are already on local authority waiting lists it would seem that the central purpose of the legislation – to stop the so-called 'fast track' into council housing by compelling homeless families to join the ordinary waiting list – is already in large measure happening. Despite its problems, the established system enjoys a broad measure of support from the local authorities. Over three-quarters of authorities in the study by Butler *et al.* (1994) described the current legislation as 'quite successful'. Their two principal complaints about it were, first, the definition of priority need which excludes single people and couples without children, and second, that officers are given too much discretion, leading to discrepancies between authorities, an over-use of appeals procedures and costly court cases. The 1997 system will do nothing to meet these problems. *New* layers of litigation are implicit within the statute over such questions as the new eligibility rules (as we have seen, already subject to challenge), the insertion of 'other good reason' into the intentionality clauses and, of course, the definition of 'other suitable accommodation'. Disaggregating the now well-established administrative procedures for dealing with homeless applicants from the rest of the allocation and selection procedures is a potentially complex bureaucratic problem, and means that, in effect, authorities will have to have two systems, one dealing with the 'normal' waiting-list allocations and a parallel but clearly separate track for the homeless.

Part VII of the Housing Act 1996 is an historical throwback. Under the new system the punitive attitude of the Poor Law workhouse is re-kindled in modern guise as the hostels and residual private rental accommodation to which homeless families will now be destined, and with no certainty of long-term help. More even than this is the fact that the language and prejudices of the Poor Law (truthfully never far from the surface of the 1977 system) are set to recover the lost ground of twenty years. The burden of challenging this falls on the political system and it is an indictment of it rather than the law that the shameful legacy of the Poor Law is to be carried forward into the twenty-first century.

NOTES

1 The author wishes to express his gratitude to his friend and colleague Professor David Hughes (School of Law at De Montfort University) for his assistance in the preparation of this chapter.

Chapter 3

Theorising homelessness
Contemporary sociological and feminist perspectives[1]

Joanne Neale

This chapter examines the relationship between homelessness and social theory and is based on a number of key assumptions. First, although theory will not directly explain the development of policy or provision for homeless people, it is an important consideration which should not be ignored. Second, various theories of homelessness which have influenced policy and provision for homeless people to date are in many respects inadequate. Third, a more comprehensive theoretical understanding of the needs and circumstances of homeless people cannot guarantee improvements in provision, but good practice is more likely to result from good theory than from poor or from inadequate explanations. Increasing our understanding of the relationship between homelessness and social theory is, therefore, an important objective.

The chapter does not attempt to devise a single, new, all-encompassing theory of homelessness but rather highlights aspects of theory which might prove enlightening. To this end, the first section provides an overview of some common theories of homelessness and shows how these have influenced provision for people who are homeless to date. The second section provides a feminist critique of such theories, but concludes that feminist arguments are not in themselves unproblematic. Inspired by more recent feminist debates, the third section considers the potential of postmodern and poststructuralist thinking for developing a more comprehensive understanding of homelessness. Postmodernist and poststructuralist arguments are found to be enlightening, but also constrained by various critical weaknesses. Consequently, the notion of 'structuration' (Giddens 1979, 1984) is introduced. The chapter concludes by suggesting how the theory considered in the preceding sections might be applied to policy and practice responses to homelessness.

EXISTING THEORIES OF HOMELESSNESS

The theoretical explanations of homelessness which have informed policies and provision for homeless people to date have tended to be implicit and contradictory rather than explicit and consistent. Nevertheless, various common themes recur. Thus, homelessness has often been explained simplistically and somewhat atheoretically as either a housing or a welfare problem, caused by either structural or individual factors (Johnson *et al.* 1991). A structural explanation of homelessness looks beyond the individual and considers broader social and economic factors – such as the role of housing systems and markets and the availability of housing. An appropriate response, according to this model, requires intervention on a broad societal scale. This might include subsidies to the housing market or the direct provision of temporary or permanent accommodation.

Individual (or agency) explanations of homelessness divide into two strands. According to the first, individuals are considered responsible for their homelessness and hence guilty and blameworthy. Individuals believed to be homeless for these reasons are often associated with the stereotypes of deviants, dossers, alcoholics, vagrants and tramps. This is a victim-blaming explanation, usually invoking only a minimalist response such as the provision of very basic accommodation. The second strand of agency explanations maintains that people become homeless because of personal failure or inadequacy for which they cannot be held entirely responsible. These individuals are considered to be in need of humanitarian assistance, usually casework or psychiatric treatment, in order for them to function. A minimalist response is here usually deemed insufficient (Johnson *et al.* 1991).

Two other commonly occurring themes in theorising homelessness are the notions of 'deserving' and 'undeserving'. 'Structure' and 'agency', 'deserving' and 'undeserving' are not, however, unrelated. Where homelessness has been interpreted as a function of structural factors beyond individual control, homeless people have often been considered deserving of assistance. Conversely, where individuals have been deemed responsible for their homelessness, they have frequently been considered less worthy of support. Historically, individual explanations of homelessness have tended to predominate. Responses to homelessness have, therefore, often consisted of minimal and punitive forms of support which have emphasised the concept of less eligibility and excluded all but the most 'deserving' and 'desperate' of people (Clapham *et al.* 1990; Evans 1991).

For example, the casual wards and workhouses provided by the Poor Law authorities offered only the most primitive and punitive forms of shelter for the destitute. Similarly, the night refuges established by voluntary organisations during the second half of the nineteenth century encouraged individuals to be responsible citizens, to stand on their own two feet and to fight their weakness of character. Thus, hostels which were basic in standards and amenities, but provided support and supervision, evolved in response to the common belief that homelessness was related to personal problems and homeless people were in some way responsible for their predicament (Evans 1991).

The National Assistance Act 1948 placed statutory responsibility for homeless people on welfare, rather than housing, departments. This confirmed homelessness as a welfare, rather than a housing, problem. The traditional pathological social work approach to homelessness, with its emphasis on individual counselling and casework, was reaffirmed. Moreover, by only offering 'temporary' assistance where circumstances were 'unforeseen' (that is unintentional) the principle of less eligibility was simultaneously retained (Clapham *et al.* 1990). This pathology model of homelessness, which stressed the deviant characteristics of homeless individuals rather than issues such as housing shortage, prevailed throughout the 1960s.

During the 1970s and 1980s, links were increasingly made between homelessness and the wider structural issue of the availability of housing. An acceptance that many homeless households required little if any support, just a permanent home of their own, also grew. Reflecting this, the Housing (Homeless Persons) Act 1977 shifted responsibility away from welfare services and onto housing departments for the first time. Interestingly, however, the notions of deservingness and less eligibility remained enshrined in the legislation. Indeed, according to British law people are still only accepted for rehousing and hence implicitly considered 'deserving' of state assistance if they fulfil the criteria of being in priority need and are unintentionally homeless.

Today the poor conditions of much temporary accommodation provided by housing departments in response to housing needs frequently exacerbate health, work and other personal problems, and even generate them for many individuals who previously were without them (Clapham *et al.* 1990). Furthermore, recent research (for example, Niner 1989; Evans 1991; Elam 1992; Anderson *et al.* 1993; Bines 1994; Pleace 1995; this volume) has shown that many homeless people do have needs for support in accommodation and, hence, do require more than just permanent rehousing. The ability of housing departments to deal with homelessness in isolation is then perhaps questionable. This poses a dilemma. Are attempts to define homelessness as either a housing or a welfare problem, or as a structural or an agency issue, with individuals either deserving or blameworthy, turning full circle? Alternatively, are explanations of homelessness perhaps not so simple after all? The remainder of this chapter will argue the case for the latter.

CRITIQUES OF EXISTING THEORY

Throughout much of the post-war period a prevailing welfare consensus, sustained by a Fabian-dominated tradition of social administration, provided a basis for critiques of social inequality and a logic for establishing potentially corrective and transformative policy. There was, in other words, a collective commitment to welfare. Changes, it was assumed, could be effected unproblematically by ideas, or by the presentation of evidence, or by rational debate (Williams 1989). Consistent with this doctrine, homelessness could be explained, the needs of homeless people quantified and suitable accommodation provided in response (dependent only on the political will of those in power).

By the 1970s, however, many of the beliefs which had informed such consensus began to fade. It no longer seemed possible to agree on the normative definitions of values such as truth, justice and deservingness, which had previously underpinned welfare provision (Hewitt 1992). Likewise, it no longer seemed possible to quantify exactly what constituted poverty, need or homelessness, or to explain precisely how such circumstances arose. As a result, rational responses to quantifiable problems, such as homelessness, no longer seemed possible. Likewise, policies and provision for homeless people, based on simplistic dualistic distinctions such as deserving or undeserving, in need or not in need, homeless or not homeless, no longer seemed adequate. Although the feminist debates evolving during the 1970s and 1980s did not provide a thoroughly developed alternative theoretical framework for understanding society and social problems such as homelessness, they clearly highlighted some of the inadequacies of the existing simplistic dualistic explanations discussed above. Furthermore, they are helpful in establishing how it might be possible to move the debate forward.

Feminist critiques

In the 1960s and 1970s, the women's movement began to ask fundamental questions about the bureaucratic control and the professional authority which it saw throughout much of the welfare state (Wilson 1977; Williams 1989). Contributing to this debate, feminist critiques of housing policy and provision argued that women had frequently been neglected or marginalised in much contemporary housing-related thought, policy and practice. In respect of this, access to housing, housing design, and the meaning of the home and homelessness elicited particular criticism (Watson 1984, 1986, 1987, 1988; Watson and Austerberry 1986; Banion and Stubbs 1986; Pascall 1991; Munro and Madigan, 1993). Women, it was argued, had frequently been powerless to define their own housing needs or to house themselves independently from a man. This was because patriarchal assumptions were embedded in housing production, allocation and consumption in each of the tenures (Watson 1987 and 1988; Banion and Stubbs 1986). Such inequalities were, moreover, underpinned by gender inequalities in income resulting from the labour market (Clapham *et al.* 1990).

Feminists argued that the meaning of home was bound up with ideas of companionate marriage, children and shared activities, but such socially and historically specific interpretations stigmatised and ghettoised those who did not conform to this pattern (for example, gay and lesbian families, lone-parent families, single-person households, and those who lived in residential homes). Indeed, even within the nuclear family home-owning household, men more often actually 'owned' the property and 'controlled' the finances, whilst women were left to 'manage' often limited resources (Pahl 1982; Graham 1984; Watson 1988; Munro and Madigan 1993). The uncritical acceptance of a harmonious image of family life, meanwhile, failed to reveal the miseries of many housewives and the extent of family violence (Barrett and McIntosh 1982).

According to Watson and Austerberry, women's domestic role results in a specific meaning of the home for women (Watson and Austerberry 1986). Munro and Madigan (1993) also concluded that privacy, and by implication 'home', have very different meanings for men, women and children. This, Munro and Madigan suggested, is caused by differences in work patterns, economic independence and social expectations. Historically, women have tended to spend more time than men in the home, and this, combined with domestic labour, has meant that women have been more likely than men to feel that their personal identity is inextricably linked to it. Similarly, women's homelessness is more fully understood in the context of both the sexual division of labour and ideological pressures on women to conform to their role of housewife and mother (Watson and Austerberry 1986). Because the domestic and privatised sphere may constitute the only area of control and influence in the lives of some women, the loss of accommodation considered to be home may have profound implications in terms of feelings of lost control over life more generally.

As Watson argued, women's domestic role and economic dependence within the family has meant that a woman has been less likely than a male partner to have the resources to make alternative accommodation arrangements, if circumstances within the home are unsatisfactory. Likewise, if the house is physically in a poor condition, the woman (as domestic labourer spending most time in the home) has been more susceptible to any resultant problems. A woman may thus be located at a different stage along a home-to-homelessness continuum from her male partner and that stage will more likely be nearer the homelessness end of the scale (Watson 1984).

Such theorising suggests that one individual in a household may be considered homeless, whilst another is not (Watson 1984). Moreover, it is not possible simply to say that people are either homeless or not. As Watson (1988) argued, traditional definitions, which conceive of homelessness as a predominantly male problem, confined to male vagrants sleeping on park benches, are inadequate. Women's homelessness is frequently experienced, manifested and tackled in different ways from men's and discourses of female homelessness must, therefore, also differ. In this way, feminist arguments have revealed the need for a more relative and flexible approach to defining homelessness. Simultaneously, this would bring a greater recognition of the plight of the many individuals whose homelessness has in various ways been less public and, hence, more concealed.

Feminist analyses have thus drawn attention to many of the limitations of existing theories of homelessness and welfare and have highlighted some of the shortcomings of existing policy and practice responses. Such critiques are, however, not in themselves unproblematic. This is because welfare policy has often supported women and women have frequently promoted and defended forms of state provision. Indeed, public-sector housing is the chief resource of women without male breadwinners, and women, as mothers, have frequently been given a special claim to local authority housing (Pascall 1991). Likewise, the provision of social housing, combined with housing benefit, has to a significant degree broken the link between earning money and securing accommodation. This has also increased women's chances of gaining access to accommodation, other than by joining households economically dependent upon a male breadwinner (Watson 1986; Clapham *et al.* 1990).

Additionally, feminist critiques have been in danger of producing a 'women and' approach to issues. This is the tendency to append women as a separate category with different needs from everyone else. Implicitly this portrays men's lives as the norm and women's lives as all the same. Categorising homeless women together in this way, as one homogeneous group, ignores the diversity of women's experiences, but also assumes that specific characteristics are inherently male or female and not susceptible to change (Watson and Austerberry 1986; Watson 1988). The position of women *vis-á-vis* state welfare provision varies between individuals and between groups of individuals (lone parents, single young women, older women and so on) across societies and across cultures. Women's lives, living arrangements and accommodation patterns are also susceptible to change over time. Women have different experiences which include differing relations to the home, to the family and to homelessness. Likewise, they have different relations to tenure forms and to tenure experiences in different social and spatial contexts (Banion and Stubbs 1986). Because the feminist critiques presented in the previous section cannot account for such variations, they are in danger of being monocultural and ahistorical.

During the 1970s, feminist theorising based itself on the notion of an essential 'we' of womanhood. This was on the grounds that essential differences existed between women and men and all women shared common interests, as women, oppressed by all men (Ramazanoğlu 1989). Just as social policy tended to draw upon simplistic dualisms to explain complex phenomena, so feminist theory frequently attempted to explain women's diverse and complex experiences by drawing upon a range of unsophisticated binary oppositions. These included male/female, public/private, work/home, production/reproduction and subject/object.

A critique of welfare and housing based on essentialist notions of womanhood and simplistic binary oppositions may uncover many of the disadvantages and inequalities which women face, but can ignore the complexity and ambiguity of the relationship of individual women to welfare institutions and provision. It is also in danger of simply inserting women as objects of study and passive victims of circumstances beyond their control. This can be disempowering as it ignores the fact that women are active participants in negotiable processes (Watson 1988). Increasingly, however, feminism has recognised and attempted to deal with such issues (Segal 1987; Weedon 1987; Ramazanoğlu 1989).

Since the 1970s, differences between women have increasingly come to the fore. These have included differences of race, gender, age, class, nationality, imperialism, sexual orientation, values, culture, politics and individual biography. Recognition of these differences, and of the diversity of women's experiences, has meant acknowledging the power which some women hold and exercise over others and the political and economic interests shared by some women with some men (Ramazanoğlu 1989). Women are not simply passive victims constrained to the private sphere of the home, nor are all women oppressed by all men in all spheres in the same way. Their personal situations are, nevertheless, not impervious to public factors such as laws, state policies, employment structures and ideologies. Lives may, in other words, be circumscribed and channelled by ideologies and structural factors, but they are not necessarily predetermined or controlled by them and change is possible.

The task more recently for feminism has thus been to acknowledge the ways in which women's lives are structured by public factors, but without constructing women as homogeneous, powerless, unthinking, unquestioning victims and, hence, denying their agency. To this end, it is necessary to reconsider the issues of difference, individuality, subjectivity, and personal experiences, but without losing sight of shared gendered experiences. In confronting issues of consensus, difference, structure, agency and other simplistic binary oppositions and dualisms, the questions facing feminist critiques of society and social problems are, in many respects, no different from those discussed above. The section to follow, therefore, considers the possibility of developing a more comprehensive theoretical understanding of homelessness which includes all people, regardless of gender or other personal differences.

NEW PERSPECTIVES ON HOMELESSNESS

Postmodernism and poststructuralism

A structuralist approach to issues contends that underlying structures are known to cause events. As a result, it is believed that general conceptual frameworks can be discovered and analysed and, subsequently, integrated and coherent theory developed. As discussed earlier, the consensus politics of the early social administrators was premised on a belief in the possibility of such reasoned and rational theory and response. Thus homelessness could be explained, the needs of homeless people quantified and suitable accommodation provided by the state in response. Feminist critiques have challenged such assumptions. Similarly, postmodernism and poststructuralism reject such beliefs.

In practice, much postmodernist and poststructuralist theory has been deconstructive in character. It has emphasised fluidity and contingency and sought to challenge and to override some of the hierarchical binary oppositions and power configurations of western culture (Barrett and Phillips 1992). According to postmodernity, knowledge cannot be based on any sure foundations of reasoning. Knowledge is, rather, characterised by a plurality of rationalities and, hence, provides little basis for secure political and moral judgement and firm governance (Hewitt 1992). Assumptions about causality are challenged because there can be no single oppressive force (neither capitalism nor patriarchy) and no single solution to any predefined social problem.

Consistent with such reasoning, analyses of power should proceed from a localised, specific and particular level (Pringle and Watson 1992). Thus, rather than search from some grand theory of power, it is preferable to focus on more immediate and smaller power structures and the points where these manifest themselves as day-to-day injustices. This shift away from a search for binary power configurations and grand theory helps to explain why many of the dualisms previously considered (such as male/female, subject/object, public/private, structure/agency, in need/not in need, deserving/not deserving, and housed/homeless) have proved less than satisfactory. The work of both Foucault (1979) and the feminist poststructuralist Weedon (1987) can now illustrate this more clearly.

Foucault (1979) does not accept that there is any one class using a particular ideology to dominate the rest of society. For him there is no global manifestation of power. Power is, rather, ubiquitous and diffuse and occurs at local points as 'micro-powers'. These micro-powers operate through normalising and individuating judgements which are designed to maintain existing power configurations in order to sustain their own 'regimes of truth'. In this respect, Foucault's work exhibits shades of functionalism. Explanations of homelessness will tend to emphasise the deviancy of homeless individuals and focus on the need to 'normalise' them. Examples of this would include attempts to rehabilitate individuals 'without a settled way of life', or efforts to 'treat' or to 'reform' them through social work intervention.

Foucault, nevertheless, retains an optimistic hope that political 'resistance' can emerge (Hewitt 1992). Change will not occur by transforming the whole at once, but injustices can be 'resisted' at the particular power points where they manifest themselves. In order to make any improvements in the lives of homeless people one does not, in other words, have to begin by eradicating all homelessness; smaller and more localised changes can also be highly effective. For example, homeless people might demand and receive a more efficient service which treats them with greater respect. Likewise, hostel residents might secure greater rights and control over the running of their accommodation or greater choice over their daily lives within it. Foucault does not attribute unqualified agency to individuals, but his emphasis on the possibility of resistance suggests that there is more scope for individual action, and hence change, than allowed for by a rigidly structural analysis. Moreover, because resistance can occur at different points, or levels, there may be a myriad of ways of challenging social inequalities. This helps to overcome the limitations of simplistic theories of binary divisions and dualisms discussed previously.

Relating these local resistances to wider structural issues, the feminist poststructuralist Weedon (1987) also contends that resistance and oppression occur at numerous different levels. Weedon maintains that the subject (for example, the homeless person) is a thinking, feeling, social agent, who is capable of resistance and reflection and is central both to the process of political change and to preserving the *status quo*. The subject cannot, however, be reduced to a conscious, knowing, unified, rational subject, the kind of sovereign individual who is commonly defended within liberal thought and social administration. This is because power relations such as patriarchy, capitalism and imperialism are structural and exist in institutions and social practices (such as housing systems).

Subjectivity, according to Weedon, is more accurately understood as a site of disunity and conflict. This, she argues, may explain why people act in ways which appear contrary to their interests. It also begins to transcend the simple structure-versus-agency analysis of personal circumstances and social problems discussed earlier. The individual is socially constituted within a multiplicity of discourses, and these compete for meaning and frequently conflict. At any given historical moment there are only a finite number of such discourses in circulation and the choices and innovations an individual is capable of are limited by the discourses which constitute her and the society in which she lives. Because only a limited range of 'obvious' or 'natural' choices are offered to society's members, most forms of social control operate on the basis of 'consent' and 'acceptance' rather than 'coercive power'.

Complementing this more complex theoretical approach to subjectivity and power, the postmodernist and poststructuralist focus on language, and the deconstruction of meaning also contributes to a better understanding of homelessness. Simultaneously, however, this process of deconstruction reveals some critical weaknesses inherent in the postmodernist argument. This is because the very broad range of meanings which can be attributed to such concepts as 'home' and 'homelessness' are revealing, but also limit their explanatory or prescriptive use.

Home, for example, implies more than just any kind of shelter. It is associated with material conditions and standards, privacy, space, control, personal warmth, comfort, stability, safety, security, choice, self-expression, and physical and emotional well-being (Watson and Austerberry 1986). Such criteria change according to the household involved, according to the individuals within it, and according to the prevailing economic, social and political climate. No single definition of the home can be considered absolute, because meaning is relative and varies historically across different regions and/or societies (Watson and Austerberry 1986; Saunders and Williams 1988).

The home is, however, more than a socio-spatial system. There is an ideological content, as well as a material base, to the notion of home. Thus, Gurney (1990) sees the home as an ideological construct, located simply 'where the heart is'. Somerville (1992), meanwhile, argues that there is no clear demarcation between real and ideal meanings of home and homelessness. Home for each individual is shaped to some extent by that person's ideal understanding of the concept, or by their beliefs about what constitutes a home. So, individuals can be roofless and yet maintain that they are not home-less because their home is on the streets. Similarly, people may have a very good material standard of accommodation, but nevertheless consider themselves to be homeless.

Such vague definitions, focusing only on subjective experience and relativity, are clearly in danger of ceasing to have any signifi-cance or any impact (Watson and Austerberry 1986). Questions must then be posed. What exactly is homelessness? How can it ever be understood, other than through subjective experience? And what role does that leave for state intervention? For social policy such ambi-guities are clearly problematic. If policy cannot even define home-lessness, how can it hope to provide for homeless people? Furthermore, if experience is 'only' expressed in private and personal terms, without a public language or understanding, causes can lose their political force and social policy becomes divested of any poten-tial for collective action (Hewitt 1992). It is at this point that the focus on deconstruction within postmodernist and poststructuralist analyses becomes unhelpful.

The postmodernist argument can, in other words, be taken too far (Walby 1992). Definitions and meanings can be deconstructed so rigorously that they lose all significance and potential for practical action. Similarly, by focusing only on subjective experience and agency the power of social structures (such as capitalism, patri-archy, imperialism or even home ownership) can be dispersed so widely that all political force is dissipated. Potent social forces do exist and being homeless is to lose a stake in several of them. Like-wise, in spite of definitional complexities, home and homelessness are also real. The inherent tendency to total subjectivity, relativity and irrationality, and a primary focus on language, limit the use of postmodernism and poststructuralism, but do not negate them entirely. Indeed, aspects of postmodernism and poststructuralism can usefully be retained and used in conjunction with the concept of 'structuration' (Giddens 1979, 1984) to important practical effect.

Structuration

Like Foucault and Weedon, Giddens (1979, 1984) considers the rela-tionship between structural and individual power relations and also attempts to overcome any simplistic division between the two. Unlike Foucault and Weedon, Giddens does not, however, focus on the role of language and his approach cannot be classified as postmodernist. He rather proposes the notion of 'structuration' as an alternative way out of the structure-versus-agency dichotomy. According to 'structuration', society does not determine individual behaviour, but nor do individuals simply create society. 'Structure' and 'action' (agency) are, rather, intimately related and neither can exist independently of the other. Structures make social action possible, but it is social action that creates those very structures.

Giddens maintains that power is a two-way process and that all individuals, even those who seem to be without much control and authority (such as homeless people), have some power and ability to resist (Giddens 1979). Agents do not have to behave in fixed ways. They are able to reflect on, and to assess, what they are doing, and they may then start to behave in new ways which alter patterns of social interaction and the social structure. Likewise, individuals may also change or reproduce society in ways that they did not deliberately intend (Giddens 1984). Consistent with Foucault and Weedon, Giddens concludes that power structures operate not so much by controlling as by placing limits upon the range of options open to an actor. Humans are limited by the power relationships which comprise social action, but it is only in very exceptional circumstances that individuals are ever completely constrained.

More sophisticated theoretical analyses of personal and public issues, such as those of Foucault (1979), Weedon (1987) and Giddens (1979, 1984), suggest that there are forces in operation which make it likely that some people, and not others, will become homeless in any given set of circumstances. Nevertheless, because personal circumstances are not predetermined and because power structures operate at different levels, there will be various ways of effecting changes to human lives. Homeless people cannot, therefore, be defined as either deserving or undeserving, entirely responsible for their problems, or victims of circumstances beyond their control. Likewise, their homelessness cannot be reduced either to a welfare or to a housing problem, caused either by structural or by individual factors alone. Homeless people are thinking, feeling, social agents with rights and responsibilities, but they are also socially constituted and, therefore, constrained in many ways. Thus they have options and choices, but these are often limited. Some suggestions as to how such theory might be applied to policy and practice responses to homelessness are now considered in the conclusion.

CONCLUSION

Homelessness cannot be explained simplistically and atheoretically. Consequently, any helpful response in the form of welfare policy or provision cannot be simplistic or atheoretical either. Homeless people occupy a range of different and shifting positions in relation to a wide variety of power structures - for example, gender, race, age, health, and the employment and the housing market. There is, in other words, no single oppressive force impinging upon their lives (Foucault 1979; Giddens 1979, 1984; Weedon 1987). Similarly, there is no single agreed cause of, and consequently no single agreed solution to, any universally accepted definition of their homelessness.

The lives of homeless people are structured by numerous public factors, but they are not predetermined by them, and change is possible. Some issues will, however, inevitably be more susceptible to alteration than others. A useful strategy in responding to homelessness will, therefore, be to identify and tackle those aspects of provision which are relatively easy to modify rather than those which are not. Although this may involve making limited small scale changes at localised levels, it does not necessarily mean losing sight of wider guiding aims and objectives. An example of this could be improving various day-to-day aspects of service delivery to homeless individuals, but without losing sight of the need to eradicate housing inequalities of all forms.

In spite of the multiple differences between homeless people, there are many common concerns for them. Issues of difference, individuality, subjectivity and personal experiences should therefore be recognised, but without neglecting shared experiences and common oppressive forces. It is, in other words, necessary to build alliances and to function co-operatively, rather than simply to work from personal needs and experiences (Ramazanoğlu 1989; Hewitt 1992). The state will have a role in defining needs and providing for homeless people, but it will not provide adequately without consulting homeless people. Moreover, if understanding is to be optimised, it will also be necessary to engage other relevant groups such as service providers, professional bodies and independent advisers. Informed and open debate between all involved parties is clearly crucial if the circumstances and needs of homeless people are to be recognised, interpreted and responded to as accurately and effectively as possible.

To conclude, individuals do not cause their own homelessness, and it is therefore unacceptable and indeed impractical to leave them to their own devices when housing and support networks fail. Homeless people are not, however, helpless victims devoid of all agency. Consequently, they have a fundamental part to play in defining their needs and in shaping the provision available to them. There are not likely to be any Utopian solutions which meet the very diverse housing and support needs of all individuals. Nevertheless, through increased communication, greater co-operation and more participation, enhanced understanding and subsequently improvements to policy and provision for homeless people seem likely to result. A more comprehensive and rigorous theoretical understanding of homelessness does not guarantee improvements in provision, but is a useful starting point for attempting to effect beneficial change. Moreover, if policy and provision are allowed to develop in an untheorised way as a response to an uncritically defined concept of homelessness, less than optimal services seem likely to persist.

NOTE

1 I have developed similar arguments in Neale, J. (1997) 'Homelessness and theory reconsidered', *Housing Studies* 12(1): 47–61.

Chapter 4

The social distribution of the experience of homelessness

Roger Burrows

This chapter attempts to answer two questions. First, how widespread is the experience of homelessness? Second, how is this experience socially distributed? It does this by offering a secondary analysis of data from the *Survey of English Housing 1994/95* (SEH).[1] The SEH is a continuous government survey which began in April 1993. It is based upon interviews with about 20,000 private households in England each year (about 5,000 per quarter). Details of the sample design, data collection, response rates and so on are given in annual reports (Green and Hansbro 1995; Green *et al.* 1996). The SEH provides an annual nationally representative sample of a good size and covers a wide range of topics relating to housing circumstances, household structure and a host of socio-economic variables.

MEASURING THE EXPERIENCE OF HOMELESSNESS

In the last quarter of 1994 and the first quarter of 1995, 9,993 heads of household were asked whether they had experienced homelessness. They were asked:

> There is a lot of discussion these days about homelessness. Can I just check, in the last ten years, would you say that you have ever been homeless?

In response to this question 433 (4.3 per cent) heads of household said that, in their view, they had been homeless at some time during the period. These 433 were then asked:

> In the last ten years have you yourself ever approached a council as homeless?

In response to this question 331 (76.4 per cent) said that they had approached a local authority in relation to their perceived homelessness. These 331 were then asked:

Were you accepted as homeless by the council?

In response to this question 252 (76.1 per cent) said that they had been accepted as homeless by a local authority.

These three questions clearly attempt to operationalise different concepts of need (Bradshaw 1972). The first question attempts to measure *felt* need (or the lay perception of need). The second question attempts to measure *expressed* need (or *felt* need turned into action). The third question attempts to measure *normative* need (or professional or legal definitions of need).

There are a number of problems with the manner in which the SEH collects data on the experience of homelessness. First, the question is only asked of individuals who are currently classified as a head of household. Therefore the data might not be representative of all individuals. It may under represent women's experience of homelessness in particular. Second, the ten-year period which the first question covers is an arbitrary one. Third, the measurement of felt need which the first question attempts to tap is essentially subjective ('would *you say* that you have ever been homeless?'). The meaning attached to this question is likely to vary significantly between different groups of people. However, to some extent *all* definitions of homelessness are subjective – including, in some circumstances, councils' definition of the law (Pleace *et al.*, this volume). Fourth, no question is asked concerning the length of time of any perceived homelessness. There is a world of difference between being without a roof for one night and being without one for a prolonged period. Some people who are inadequately housed may also regard themselves as being homeless (Pleace *et al.*, this volume). Fifth, the questions are only asked of people currently living within household settings. The data do not pick up individuals who are currently living in institutional settings such as hostels. Sixth, the data only cover heads of households in England and not the whole of Britain.[2] We need to be clear, then, that the analysis which follows is not a description of the characteristics of individuals who are currently homeless. Rather, it is an analysis of the characteristics of individuals who are currently heads of households in England who at some time in the last ten years felt themselves to be homeless for any period. Nevertheless, despite these problems the data still provide some interesting insights into the social distribution of the experience of homelessness.

THE EXPERIENCE OF HOMELESSNESS IN ENGLAND BY SELECTED CURRENT HOUSEHOLD CHARACTERISTICS

Table 4.1 shows how the responses to the three questions vary in relation to differences in the characteristics of respondents in terms of: their current age; the region in which they currently live; whether or not they currently live in an urban or a rural area; their current employment status; their ethnicity; the current composition of the household they live within; their social class; their current marital status; and the tenure of the accommodation they currently live in. These different characteristics will each be discussed in turn.

Age

There is a very clear association between the age of a head of household and the chances that they have perceived themselves to be homeless at some time in the last ten years. Almost 14 per cent of young people aged between 16 and 29, and 6 per cent of those aged between 30 and 44 have felt themselves to be homeless. After the age of 45 the chances of experiencing homelessness in the last ten years declines markedly. The experience of homelessness is thus one overwhelmingly concentrated amongst younger people. The chances that a person who has felt themselves to be homeless and has presented themselves as such to a local authority also appears to be associated with age. Of those aged 16 to 29 almost 82 per cent presented themselves as homeless. People in other age groups were less likely to have presented themselves. Of those people who presented themselves as homeless, about three-quarters were accepted as such by a local authority. This proportion varied slightly with age, with those aged between 30 and 44 being slightly more likely to be have been accepted than people in other age groups.

Region

The experience of homelessness varies significantly across the different regions of England. We have already seen that for England

Table 4.1 The experience of homelessness in England by selected current household characteristics

	N	% who have perceived themselves to be homeless in last 10 years	N	...and % of these who approached a local authority	N	...and % of these who were accepted as homeless
Age						
16–29	1,196	13.7	164	81.7	134	75.4
30–44	2,961	6.0	178	73.6	131	77.1
45–54	1,784	2.5	44	79.5	35	74.3
55–64	1,525	2.2	34	70.6	24	76.0
65–74	1,509	0.9	13	53.8	7	71.4
75+	1,018	0.0	0	—	—	—
Regions						
London	1,327	6.2	82	78.0	64	76.6
Rest of South East	1,528	3.5	53	73.6	39	82.1
South West	1,024	6.1	62	69.4	43	83.7
East Anglia	1,190	3.9	47	80.9	38	71.1
East Midlands	809	3.3	27	74.1	20	60.0
West Midlands	1,021	3.5	36	86.1	31	71.0
Yorks & Humber	1,100	4.1	45	86.7	39	79.5
North East	537	4.7	25	84.0	21	71.4
North West	1,454	3.9	56	64.3	36	77.8
Urban/Rural						
Urban	8,249	4.8	399	76.9	307	75.6
Rural	1,744	1.9	34	70.6	24	83.3

Table 4.1 (cont.)

	N	% who have perceived themselves to be homeless in last 10 years	N	. . . and % of these who approached a local authority	N	. . . and % of these who were accepted as homeless
Current employment status						
Employed full-time	5,139	3.0	153	67.3	104	68.0
Employed part-time	487	7.8	38	84.2	32	84.4
Unemployed	609	14.4	88	78.4	69	68.1
Retired	2,688	0.7	19	63.2	12	66.7
Other inactive	1,063	12.4	132	93.2	112	86.6
Ethnicity						
White	9,518	4.2	399	75.7	302	76.2
Black	164	13.4	22	90.9	20	70.0
Indian	125	2.4	3	100.0	3	100.0
Pakistani/Bangladeshi	53	3.8	2	100.0	2	100.0
Other	131	4.6	6	50.0	3	66.6
Current household structure						
Couple, no dependent children	3,614	1.5	54	68.5	37	56.8
Couple, with dependent children	2,666	4.4	117	76.9	90	81.1
Lone parent	624	19.7	123	93.5	115	87.8
Complex adult household	576	3.1	18	61.1	11	45.5
Single male	1,034	7.4	76	64.5	49	61.2
Single female	1,479	3.0	45	64.4	29	75.9

Social class of head of household

Professional	697	0.4	3	0.0	—	—
Intermediate	2,616	2.9	75	68.0	51	72.5
Skilled non-manual	1,421	4.8	68	79.4	54	75.9
Skilled manual	2,793	3.6	101	77.2	78	71.8
Semi-skilled manual	1,473	7.1	104	80.8	84	76.2
Unskilled manual	552	7.8	43	79.1	34	82.4
Armed Forces	65	3.1	2	50.0	1	100.0

Current marital status

Married	5,685	2.2	123	74.0	91	78.0
Cohabiting	687	7.4	51	76.5	39	66.7
Never married	1,272	10.7	135	75.6	102	72.5
Widowed	1,331	1.1	15	80.0	12	83.3
Separated	257	12.8	33	93.9	31	93.5
Divorced	761	10.0	76	73.7	56	75.0

Current tenure

Owns outright	2,432	0.4	10	30.0	3	0.0
Buying on mortgage	4,320	1.6	71	57.7	41	48.8
Council	1,935	11.0	211	90.5	190	86.8
Housing association	374	16.3	61	82.0	50	74.0
PRS	929	8.6	80	58.8	47	63.8

Source: SEH (1994/95), Own analysis
Note: Some figures may add up slightly incorrectly due to the effects of rounding and weighting.

as a whole the probability of experiencing homelessness at some time in the last ten years was 4.3 per cent. However, the probability of having experienced homelessness for someone currently living in Greater London or the South West of England was over a third greater than this. Over 6 per cent of household heads in these two regions stated that they had felt themselves to be homeless. The figure for those living in the North East was also greater than the national average but not significantly so. Of course this does not necessarily mean that the individuals in the sample experienced their homelessness in the regions in which they currently live. This regional variation is probably the result of a complex interaction of factors within each area: in the case of London some variation may be caused by homeless people travelling to the capital; in the South West it may be related to the constriction in social housing supply and a private rented sector (PRS) that is difficult to access due to the tourist industry (Ford *et al.* 1997).

Urban and rural areas

Regional differences in the rates at which homelessness has been experienced is overlaid with urban and rural variation.[3] Heads of household currently living in urban areas are over two and a half times more likely to have experienced homelessness in the last ten years than are heads of household currently living in rural areas. Almost 5 per cent of heads of household in urban areas claimed to have experienced homelessness, whilst in rural areas the proportion is just under 2 per cent. Those currently living in urban areas were more likely to have presented themselves as homeless to a local authority than were those living in rural areas. However, of those presenting as homeless, those living in rural areas were more likely to have been accepted as homeless by a local authority than were those currently living in urban areas. Over 83 per cent of those presenting themselves as homeless in rural areas were accepted as such by a local authority, whilst the figure for those in urban areas was just under 76 per cent.

Current employment status

Just over 14 per cent of currently unemployed heads of household had experienced homelessness, as had over 12 per cent of those who were otherwise economically inactive. Of those currently employed part-time almost 8 per cent had experienced homelessness. These figures compare with just 3 per cent of those who are currently employed full-time. Under 1 per cent of retired heads of household had experienced homelessness. The experience of homelessness is thus heavily concentrated amongst those who are currently economically inactive. For instance, the currently unemployed are almost five times more likely to have experienced homelessness than are those heads of household currently employed full-time.

Ethnicity

The experience of homelessness is greatest amongst heads of household who identify themselves as 'Black'. Almost 14 per cent of heads of household who identify themselves as such have experienced homelessness. The proportions of those experiencing homelessness amongst households with heads who identify themselves as 'Indian', 'Pakistani' or 'Bangladeshi' is below the average for the population as a whole. Although the overwhelming majority of people who have experienced homelessness are 'White', the 'risk' of having experienced this form of social exclusion is greatest amongst members of the 'Black' population. A 'Black' head of household is over three times more likely to have experienced homelessness than is a 'White' head of household.

Current household structure

Lone parents and single males are the most likely to have experienced homelessness. Almost 20 per cent of individuals who are currently lone parents (the great majority of whom are female) and over 7 per cent of men who are currently living on their own have experienced homelessness. The figure for lone parents is the highest proportion in any of the various characteristics considered here. Essentially, the data suggest that about one-fifth of all lone parents in England have, at some time, experienced a period of homelessness. The figures also show that although lone-parent households constitute only 6.2 per cent of all households, they make up 28.4 per cent of all households who have presented themselves as homeless to local authorities, and almost 36 per cent of all those accepted as such.

Social class

The experience of homelessness is profoundly related to social class. Of those who are currently classified as professionals, just 0.4 per cent have some experience of homelessness. This compares with 7.8 per cent of those currently classified in the unskilled manual occupational class category. In more general terms, the data show that those from manual social class backgrounds are about one and two-thirds times more likely to have experienced homelessness than are those from non-manual social class backgrounds. It is also interesting to note that of those classified as being in the Armed Forces, just 3.1 per cent claimed to have had some experience of homelessness. This finding strengthens the claim by Higate (this volume) that the extent of homelessness amongst ex-service personnel has perhaps hitherto been somewhat overstated.

Current marital status

Those heads of household who are single and have never married and those who are currently separated or divorced are the most likely to have experienced homelessness. About one in ten of currently single and currently divorced heads of household claim to have experienced homelessness. Amongst heads of household who are currently separated the figure is almost one in eight. The experience of homelessness is comparatively rare amongst people who are currently married or have been widowed.

Tenure of current accommodation

The experience of homelessness is rare amongst people who are currently home owners. For instance, just 1.6 per cent of current mortgagors have experienced homelessness. Heads of households with any experience of homelessness are heavily concentrated in the social rented sector and, to a slightly lesser extent, in the PRS. Some of this tenurial distribution of the experience of homelessness will be due to the statutory responsibilities of local authorities to rehouse households who are homeless and in priority need (Lowe, this volume). However, some of this tenurial distribution of the experience of homelessness will also be due to the concentration of households with characteristics which predispose them to this experience within the social rented sector – youth, economic exclusion, minority ethnic group membership, manual social class backgrounds and so on.

MODELLING THE CHANCES THAT A HEAD OF HOUSEHOLD HAS EXPERIENCED HOMELESSNESS

The data in Table 4.1 have allowed us to form a relatively clear picture of the social distribution of the experience of homelessness in England by considering the impact of a selection of different socio-economic characteristics in turn. However, we can considerably extend the analysis by considering what the impact of different combinations of factors has on the chances of having experienced homelessness. However, in order to do this we need to undertake some fairly simple multivariate statistical analysis. Our task is to try and decipher what combination of attributes best predict that a head of household will have experienced homelessness. In this way we shall be able to establish a model able to predict what the chances are that a head of household with any given combination of socio-economic attributes will have experienced homelessness. In order to do this, a logistic regression analysis was carried out on the data. Logistic regression establishes the effect that a range of different variables (such as those already considered above) have on the chances (or odds) of a head of household having experienced homelessness. Unlike bivariate analyses, which compare the effect of one variable on the chances of having experienced homelessness, logistic regression examines the effect of a range of variables simultaneously and thus allows us to gauge the relative effect of different variables. The results from this are shown in Table 4.2.

Bivariate results

The first column shows the impact that the nine variables already considered above have on the odds[4] of experiencing homelessness when each is considered independently. Some of them have been simplified in order to demonstrate the significant contrasts between categories more clearly, and age has been entered as a cardinal variable rather than an ordinal one. These results are simply another way of expressing the results already discussed. For the eight variables which are categorical, the odds of experiencing homelessness for different categories within each variable is compared to an arbitrary 'reference' category. So, for instance, compared to living in an urban area the odds of experiencing homelessness are decreased by a factor of 0.39 for heads of household living in a rural area (sig. at $p < 0.001$). Or, to take another example, compared to being employed full-time those heads

Table 4.2 Logistic regression models predicting experience of homelessness

Variable	Exponentiated bivariate parameters	Exponentiated parameters for 'best-fitting model'
Base odds	Varies	0.12***
Age (continuous)	0.93***	0.94***
Area		
Rest of England	1.00	1.00
London	1.63***	1.09
Rest of South East	0.89	1.13
South West	1.60**	2.56***
Urban/Rural		
Urban	1.00	1.00
Rural	0.39***	0.63*
Current employment status		
Employed full-time	1.00	—
Employed part-time	2.76***	—
Unemployed	5.50***	—
Retired	0.24***	—
Other inactive	4.62***	—
Ethnicity		
White	1.00	—
Black	3.53***	—
Indian	0.56	—
Pakistani/Bangladeshi	1.34	—
Other	0.84	—

Current household structure

All others	1.00	—
Couples, with dependent children	2.17***	—
Lone parents	11.64***	—
Single male	3.81***	—

Social class of head of household

Professional	1.00	—
Intermediate	6.74**	—
Skilled non-manual	11.47***	—
Skilled manual	8.56***	—
Semi-skilled manual	17.51***	—
Unskilled manual	19.28***	—

Current marital status

Married	1.00	1.00
Cohabiting	3.63***	1.23
Never married	5.41***	1.28
Widowed	0.52*	1.06
Seperated/divorced	5.42***	2.26***

Current tenure

Owner occupation	1.00	1.00
Council	10.13***	8.04***
Housing association	16.05***	10.97***
PRS	7.76***	3.34***

Table 4.2 (cont.)

Variable	Exponentiated bivariate parameters	Exponentiated parameters for 'best-fitting model'
Interaction		
Not	—	1.00
Employed part-time*		
couple, dependent children	—	1.95
lone parent	—	1.29
single male	—	1.30
Unemployed*		
couple, dependent children	—	1.74*
lone parent	—	0.99
single male	—	2.14**
Retired*		
couple, dependent children	—	4.04
lone parent	—	8.51
single male	—	1.38
Other inactive*		
couple, dependent children	—	1.74
lone parent	—	1.40
single male	—	2.65***

Source: SEH (1994/95). Own analysis

Notes:
For the 'best-fitting' model, the R_L^2 is 25.65 per cent and the model chi-square is 911.058 sig. at $p < 0.001$.

*p < 0.05
**p < 0.01
***p < 0.001

of household who are currently unemployed are 5.5 times more likely to have experienced homelessness (p < 0.001). For variables such as age, which are measured at a cardinal level, the estimate gives an indication of the rate at which the odds of the experience of homelessness increases or decreases with each additional unit change in the variable. So, for instance, the figure of 0.93 means that as age increases the odds of experiencing homelessness decrease by a factor of 0.93 per year (p < 0.001).

The great advantage of logistic regression is that one can easily move beyond this simple bivariate form of analysis and control for the influences of all of the other variables simultaneously. The final column in Table 4.2 shows what happens when all of the variables considered in the first column are considered simultaneously and then the combination of variables which best predicts the experience of the homelessness are selected. In essence, the model which results is the one which maximises our ability to predict correctly that a head of household with a given combination of attributes has experienced homelessness. This final 'best-fitting' model (to use the argot) contains seven of the original nine variables considered. Five of them enter the final model on their own and two enter as a complex 'interaction' effect. What does the model mean?

The 'best-fitting' model

The model suggests that the age of a head of household, the area in which they currently live, their current marital status, the tenure of their current accommodation, their employment status and the composition of the household within which they currently live will allow us to explain 25.65 per cent of the variation in the odds of a head of household experiencing homelessness over the last ten years.[5]

The base odds figure of 0.12 is the estimated odds that someone with the combination of 'reference' category characteristics has experienced homelessness. That is someone living in the 'rest of England', in an urban settlement, who is married and living as a couple with no dependent children, living in owner-occupied accommodation and employed full-time. The model shows how this estimated odds figure is increased or decreased if these characteristics are altered.

The figure for age of 0.94 (p < 0.001) shows that the influence of age continues to decrease the odds of homelessness even after the influence of all the other variables in the model are controlled for. On average, for every additional year an individual ages their odds of having experienced homelessness decreases by a factor of 0.94 (that is, the odds are reduced by about 6 per cent per annum).

The influence of region is altered when controlled for by the other variables in the model. The increased odds of experiencing homelessness in London disappears. However, the increased odds is strengthened for the South West. This means that when differences in age structure, urban/rural settlements, current marital status, current tenure, employment status and household composition are considered, the only region in England which appears to increase the odds of experiencing homelessness in its own right is the South West. The increased odds in London was simply a by-product of the influence of some of these other factors acting through the area.

The urban/rural differences in the experiences of homelessness are maintained when all of the variables are controlled for, but at a much lower level. When all of the other variables in the model are controlled for, the odds of having experienced homelessness are reduced by a factor of 0.63 ($p < 0.05$) for those living in rural settlements compared to those living in urban areas.

The influence on having experienced homelessness of current employment status does not appear in the model in its own right. Any influence that it has only occurs in combination with particular types of household structure – single males and couples with dependent children. For single males the odds of having experienced homelessness are significantly increased if they are unemployed or otherwise economically inactive ($p < 0.001$). For couples with dependent children the odds are significantly increased if the head of household is currently unemployed ($p < 0.05$).

The influence of ethnicity on the odds of homelessness does not appear in the 'best-fitting' model. Although it appears that those heads of household who identify themselves as 'Black' are significantly more likely to have experienced homelessness, this increased propensity disappears when the other variables in the model are controlled for. Thus, rather than it being ethnicity *per se* which increases the odds, it is more likely that it is other characteristics which 'Black' heads of household possess which account for the association – factors such as living in an urban area, being economically inactive, living within a particular type of household, living within a particular type of tenure and so on.

The current household structure, like current employment status, does not appear in the 'best-fitting' model on its own, but only in combination with current employment status. The nature of this 'interaction' effect has been discussed above.

The impact of the social class of the head of household on the odds of experiencing homelessness also drops out of the 'best-fitting' model when all of the other variables in the model are controlled for. Thus, rather than it being social class *per se* which increases the odds of homelessness, it is the characteristics associated with different social classes which increase the odds. Being in lower social classes increases the likelihood that someone will be exposed to the other risk factors associated with homelessness. In particular, it is likely that the variations across social classes which appear when considered within the bivariate model are, in actuality, by-products of the effects of tenure, current employment status and possibly also current household structure on the odds of experiencing homelessness.

The influence of current marital status is maintained in the 'best-fitting model but the nature of the association is altered when the other variables in the model are controlled for. Only heads of household who are currently divorced or separated are significantly more likely to have experienced homelessness compared to someone who is currently married.

Finally, the impact of current tenure on the odds of experiencing homelessness is maintained even after all of the other variables in the model are controlled for. Compared to heads of household currently in owner occupation, the model predicts that those currently living in housing association accommodation are almost eleven times more likely to have experienced homelessness, those in local authority accommodation over eight times more likely and those currently living in the PRS over three times more likely.[6]

CONCLUSIONS

Overall the SEH data estimate that some 4.3 per cent of heads of household in England have experienced homelessness at some time in the last ten years. However, only 3.3 per cent presented themselves as homeless to a local authority and only 2.5 per cent were accepted as such by a local authority. Crudely, then, the data suggest that if we take the number of local authority homeless acceptances as an indicator of the prevalence of homelessness in England, this figure will underestimate the numbers of heads of household who perceived themselves to be homeless by a factor of about 50 per cent.

Not surprisingly, the analysis has also clearly demonstrated that the experience of homelessness is not evenly distributed across the population. Rather, it is very clearly socially patterned. This social patterning has been examined in three different ways. First, the proportions of heads of households with different socio-economic characteristics who have experienced homelessness were examined. Second, the odds that heads of households with given socio-economic characteristics have experienced homelessness were examined. Third, a multivariate statistical model was fitted to the data in order to ascertain the combination of characteristics which best predicted that a head of household has experienced homelessness at some time in the last ten years.

The combination of characteristics which produced the highest odds of experiencing homelessness were: being young; living in the South West; living in an urban settlement; being divorced or separated; living in housing association accommodation; and being a single male who is currently economically inactive. At the other extreme, the combination of characteristics which produced the lowest odds of experiencing homelessness were: being old; living in the provinces (but outside the South West); living in a rural area; being married; living in owner-occupation; being employed full-time; and living in a couple without dependent children.

There is then a considerable degree of social and demographic distance between those who have and those who have not experienced homelessness. However, although the odds of experiencing homelessness are low for the majority of people and the direct physical and psychological impact of homelessness effects only about 4 per cent (some 2 million people) of the population, there are strong arguments which suggest that, in actuality, homelessness effects all of us. As Wilkinson (1996) has recently argued, the health and well-being of the whole population is increasingly undermined by a social system which invokes insecurity and is so grossly unequal. The mechanisms by which *relative* inequalities are translated into *direct* impacts upon the health and well-being of us all are complex. However, in the case of homelessness the following quotation from a study of youth homelessness by Pat Carlen gives at least a flavour of one of the mechanisms by which the experience of homelessness by a minority has an impact upon us all:

So often have we been told that the market gives and the market takes away, that a hitherto unacceptable level of unemployment is necessary to bring inflation down, that the homeless on the streets can indicate to us in a very tangible way that the requisite sacrificial lambs are indeed upon the altar, that the market gods are being appeased. Even if people wanted to intervene, how could they when their own jobs have become so uncertain, when a generalized fear of risk and uncertainty, together with the prevailing ethic of individualism make it almost *immoral to care*?

(Carlen 1996: 80)

Homelessness, then, generates a wider sense of unease amongst the wider population, especially at a time of substantial economic and employment restructuring already invoking widespread feelings of insecurity.

NOTES

1 Material from the SEH was made available through the Office of National Statistics and the ESRC Data Archive with the permission of the Controller of HM Stationery Office.
2 Recent data suggest that in Scotland about 5 per cent of heads of household have experienced homelessness (Scottish Homes 1996).
3 The released SEH data files do not contain any rural/urban measures. However, a derived variable constructed by the Department of the Environment using 'mapping techniques' was released to the author for work funded by the Rural Development Commission on the housing needs of young people in rural areas (Ford *et al.* 1997). This is the variable used here. The original measure indicates if a household lives in one of three different settlement types: a 'rural settlement', defined as any settlement with a population of under 1,000 in 1991; a 'semi-rural settlement', defined as any settlement with a population of between 1,000 and 9,999 in 1991; and an 'urban settlement', defined as any settlement with a population of 10,000 or more in 1991. Here 'rural' and 'semi-rural' settlements have been collapsed into one category.
4 Those familiar with the mathematics of horse racing will recognise the odds of an event to be simply another way of expressing a probability that it will occur. The odds of an event is given by $p/(1-p)$ where p is the probability of an event occurring. As Prior (1995) has recently pointed out, in this highly individualistic age there is a widespread tendency to attach probabilities, odds or other indicators of risk to individuals. It is as if each *individual* possesses some given predisposition towards various conditions: illness; accidents; the experience of homelessness. This is, of course, a nonsense. Probabilities can only ever be understood in terms of *collective* social properties. In what follows it is important to bear this in mind. Although the language used may sometimes indicate otherwise, the odds associated with the characteristics of any given collective social group should not be imputed to any single individual or

household.

5 The level of the predictive power of models in the social and policy sciences tends, in general, to be low. In most cases we are less interested in how well we can predict phenomena than we are in trying to establish which factors significantly increase or decrease the odds of some event – in this case the experience of homelessness – occurring. However, having said this, in this particular instance the R_L^2 of over 25 per cent is high.

6 Some caution should be taken when interpreting these figures in terms of *relative risk*. The odds ratio is similar, but not identical, to relative risk. Further, when the prevalence of an outcome is high, logistic regression models can provide inaccurate estimates. Given this, it is perhaps better to interpret estimates for odds as if they were on an ordinal rather than a ratio scale. So, for example, although we can be confident that an exponentiated parameter estimate of 10.97 is greater than an exponentiated parameter estimate of 3.34, we cannot be quite so confident that it is 3.3 times as great (10.97/3.34).

Chapter 5

The characteristics of single homeless people in England

Peter A. Kemp

Historically, perceptions of single homelessness have often been based on stereotypical images of who such people are and why they are without a home of their own. One reason for this may be the relative lack of robust data on the subject. There are no statistically reliable figures on the number of single people who are homeless, and even the 1991 Census count of rough sleepers is widely regarded as a substantial underestimate (Pleace *et al.* this volume). For example, while the Census recorded a nil return for Birmingham, up to 60 people were thought to be sleeping rough in the city at the time (Adamczuk 1992). There are considerable methodological difficulties facing attempts to undertake representative surveys of single homeless people. In particular, there exists no readily available sampling frame for homeless people and compiling one is both time consuming and expensive. Perhaps for this reason, large-scale and methodologically robust surveys of single homeless people are relatively infrequently carried out and invariably funded by government departments.

Until recently, our knowledge of single people who are homeless was based on a Department of the Environment (DoE) funded survey completed in 1978, the results of which were published in 1982 (Drake *et al.* 1982). However, the nature of single homelessness is widely believed to have changed since that survey was carried out. For example, the number of single homeless people is thought to have increased (Deacon *et al.* 1995). There was a marked increase in the number of single people on social security living in board and lodging accommodation in the early 1980s (Conway and Kemp 1985). The late 1980s witnessed what appeared to be a substantial increase in the incidence of people sleeping rough on the streets, particularly in London but also in other towns and cities. However, in London the numbers of people sleeping rough have declined following the implementation of the government's Rough Sleepers Initiative (Randall and Brown 1996). In addition, there appeared to have been a change in the composition of the single homeless population. Many of the rough sleepers did not conform to the traditional stereotype of the White, elderly 'dosser' or 'down-and-out', but were in fact young people, including some women. Indeed, Centrepoint Soho argued that there was an increase in the number of young single homeless people in the 1980s.

This chapter draws on a survey of single homeless people which the author carried out with two colleagues while in the Centre for Housing Policy (CHP), on behalf of the DoE (Anderson et al. 1993).[1] The research was the first large-scale study of single homelessness to be commissioned by the Department since 1978. The fieldwork for the survey was undertaken in 1991, the same year as the last Census. The results of this research show the characteristics of single homeless people in the early 1990s in England.

METHODS

The survey involved structured interviews with people using hostels, night shelters and bed and breakfast (B&B) hotels and with people who were sleeping rough. In addition, group discussions were held with homeless people in a number of hostels and day centres. Full details of the methods employed in the research are set out in the report *Single Homeless People* (Anderson et al. 1993), but in brief they were as follows.

Interviews were completed with a representative sample of 1,346 people who were staying in *hostels, night shelters and B&B hotels.* The survey therefore excluded people in squats or staying at 'care of' addresses or living in insecure and unsatisfactory sharing arrangements. People who had dependent children in their care, or who had been placed in hostels or B&B hotels by a local authority housing department and had also been accepted for permanent rehousing, were also excluded from the survey.

The fieldwork was conducted in five London boroughs and five other English cities which analysis of DoE homelessness statistics, the London Hostels Directory and 1981 Census data on hostels and common lodging houses suggested had the highest incidence of homelessness.

The sample for the survey was drawn from a sampling frame of hostels, night shelters and B&B hotels known to be providing accommodation for single homeless people in the ten areas, compiled from information provided by the local authority and other local housing and welfare agencies. Details of each establishment were checked to establish their eligibility for the sampling frame and the number of bedspaces provided for, or normally used by, single homeless people. A two-stage probability sampling scheme was employed to ensure that each single homeless person in the sampling frame had an equal chance of being selected for interview. This was important because of the very wide range in the size of hostels and B&B hotels. Establishments were stratified according to the number of bedspaces provided for single homeless people, and a representative sample of establishments was drawn for each of the ten local authority areas in the study. The sample was therefore a representative sample of the occupants of bedspaces provided for single homeless people in each area. The achieved sample was then weighted for analysis to reflect the distribution of bedspaces between the ten areas. The response rate for the survey was 76 per cent.

Interviews were also completed with 507 people *sleeping rough*. These interviews involved people who used soup runs and day centres. Only people using day centres or soup runs who had slept rough on at least one night in the previous seven were included in the survey. The day-centre and soup-run surveys were conducted in the five London boroughs and in Manchester and Bristol. Information on day centres and soup runs, including details of the level of their usage by rough sleepers, was collected and used to create a sample quota and sampling interval for each location. Interviewers counted users entering the day centre or using the soup run and sampled every nth individual until the required number of interviews was completed. In total, 156 interviews were conducted at soup runs and 351 in day centres. The response rates were 79 per cent and 83 per cent respectively.

Users of soup runs and day centres were sampled separately because it was not clear at the design stage whether single homeless people using these two types of facility were similar or different. In fact, the two samples were very similar. Analysis of the survey data found that for the vast majority of variables there were no statistically significant differences ($p < 0.01$) between those who used soup runs and those who used day centres. In other words it can reasonably be concluded that the respondents came from the same population. The results for these two types of sampling point have therefore been aggregated for the analysis in this chapter.

Because of methodological differences, the results of the 1991 survey are not strictly comparable with those from the 1978 interviews by Drake *et al.* (1982). A quarter of the 521 interviews completed in 1978 were with clients of advice agencies, whereas the 1991 survey was confined to people who were either in temporary accommodation or sleeping rough. While the 1991 study sampled people using day centres and soup runs separately from those in hostels and night shelters, Drake *et al.* interviewed twenty-one people in day centres or soup runs and included these cases in their overall results. However, comparisons are possible between the hostel and B&B sample from the 1991 survey and the 1972 study by Digby (1976) of hostels and common lodging houses which was commissioned by the Department of Health and Social Security. Neither the 1972 survey nor the 1978 one involved a separate study of people sleeping rough.

DEMOGRAPHIC CHARACTERISTICS

A consistent finding of surveys of homeless people is that men are more likely to be homeless than women. The 1991 survey was no exception to this general pattern, but there was also a clear difference between the hostel and rough sleeping samples. While women were underrepresented among homeless people as a whole, they were significantly less likely to be sleeping rough than staying in hostels and B&Bs: they accounted for 23 per cent of people staying in hostels and B&Bs and only 9 per cent of people sleeping rough.

Whether women were less likely to be sleeping rough because they were more able or more willing to obtain temporary accommodation than men is not clear. At any rate, the great majority of single homeless people in 1991 were men: they accounted for 91 per cent of people sleeping rough and 77 per cent of people staying in hostels and B&Bs. By comparison, in his 1972 survey of hostels and common lodging houses, Digby (1976) found that 91 per cent were men and only 9 per cent were women. These figures suggest that there has been an increase in the proportion of homeless people in hostels who are women over this twenty-year period.

Single homeless people staying in hostels and B&Bs in the 1991 survey were significantly different from those sleeping rough not only in gender but also in age. People staying in hostels and B&Bs were more likely than rough sleepers to be either young adults or (to a lesser extent) elderly. Thus 30 per cent of people in hostels and B&Bs were under 25 years of age compared with 16 per cent of those sleeping rough. At the other extreme, 14 per cent of people in hostels and B&Bs compared with 9 per cent who were sleeping rough were aged 60 or over. However, the majority of homeless single people, particularly those sleeping rough, were middle-aged: 75 per cent of rough sleepers and 54 per cent of people in hostels and B&Bs were aged between 25 and 59.

There were significant age differences between homeless men and women, both among those staying in hostels and B&Bs and among those sleeping rough. The main difference was that women as a whole were a much younger population than men. For example, 50 per cent of women in hostels and B&Bs were aged under 25 compared with only 25 per cent of men. Among rough sleepers 44 per cent of women were aged under 25 compared with 13 per cent of men. Likewise, there were proportionately fewer women than men aged 45 or more, both among homeless people in hostels and B&Bs and among those sleeping rough (Table 5.1).

When the results for age in the 1991 survey are compared with those from Digby's 1972 survey, it is apparent that there was a large increase in the proportion of young single homeless people, and a decrease in the proportion of elderly single homeless people, over this period. As Table 5.2 shows, in 1972 only 11 per cent of men were aged under 30 years, but in 1991 the proportion was 39 per cent. At the other end of the spectrum, in 1972 Digby found that 32 per cent of men in hostels and common lodging houses were aged 60 or over, but in the 1991 survey 17 per cent were in that age group. A similar

Table 5.1 The age of single homeless people by gender

Age	People in hostels and B&Bs*		People sleeping rough*	
	Female (%)	Male (%)	Female (%)	Male (%)
16–17	12	3	11	1
18–24	38	22	33	12
25–44	31	38	36	48
45–59	12	20	13	29
60 and over	7	17	7	9
Don't know/ can't recall	1	1	—	1
Total	100	100	100	100
(Base)	(293)	(969)	(45)	(456)

Source: Single Homeless People Survey data (1991). Own analysis

Note:
* Significant at < 0.01

Table 5.2 The age of single homeless people in hostels and B&Bs, 1972 and 1991

Age	1972		1991	
	Males (%)	Females (%)	Males (%)	Females (%)
Under 30	11	24	39	67
30–39	11	13	17	12
40–49	21	14	14	6
50–59	25	13	13	8
60 and over	32	36	17	7
Total	100	100	100	100
(Base)	(1,821)	(172)	(959)	(291)

Sources: Digby, P.W. (1976) *Hostels and Lodgings for Single People*, OPCS, London: HMSO and Single Homeless People Survey data (1991). Own analysis

change was found among single homeless women in hostels. In 1972, 24 per cent of women were aged under 30, but in 1991 the figure was 67 per cent. And whereas 36 per cent of women were aged over 60 years in 1972, the corresponding figure for 1991 was only 7 per cent.

The ethnic background of homeless single people in hostels and B&Bs in the 1991 survey was significantly different from that of people sleeping rough. While 97 per cent of people sleeping rough described themselves as being White, among those in hostels and B&Bs the proportion was 73 per cent. People who were from Black and other minority ethnic groups were overrepresented among the hostel and B&B population but underrepresented among rough sleepers (Anderson *et al.* 1993). The reasons for this significant difference between the two samples are not clear and warrant further research.

A very wide variety of ethnic backgrounds was represented among people in hostels and B&Bs, but by far the most numerically important minorities were Black African or Black Caribbean people, who together accounted for 16 per cent of all single homeless people in hostels and B&Bs (see also Burrows, this volume). Ethnic origin did not feature in Digby's 1972 survey and it is possible to speculate from this silence that the incidence of homelessness among Black and other ethnic minority people has become substantial only since that date.

In the 1991 survey there was a significant gender difference in hostels and B&Bs, but not among rough sleepers, when those who described their ethnic background as White were compared with those from a minority group. Among people sleeping rough, 97 per cent of men and 98 per cent of women said their ethnic background was White. In hostels and B&Bs, by contrast, 80 per cent of men compared with only 52 per cent of women described themselves as White. Thus women from minority ethnic groups were significantly overrepresented among homeless single people in hostels and B&Bs.

ASPECTS OF DISADVANTAGE

Bines (1994; this volume) drawing on the results of the 1991 survey, has demonstrated that single homeless people suffer from worse health than the general population. Rough sleepers were significantly more likely to say they had health problems than were people in hostels and B&Bs. And among those who had health problems, a significantly larger percentage of rough sleepers compared with those in hostels and B&Bs (30 per cent and 21 per cent respectively) said that these had caused them difficulty in finding or keeping a place to live. These results illustrate how one disadvantage can exacerbate or even create another.

A high proportion of single homeless people had experience of a wide range of different types of 'institution', such as children's homes, prison, psychiatric units or hospitals, alcohol and drug units, and the Armed Forces. However, once again, people sleeping rough were significantly more likely to have had experience of institutional life than those who were staying in hostels and B&Bs (Table 5.3). It is possible that the disadvantages or other circumstances that had led people to spend time in an institution make it difficult for some of them to gain access to permanent accommodation or employment. But it is also possible that the experience of institutional living itself makes it difficult for some of those concerned to maintain a home of their own in a non-institutional setting – a form of 'domestic deskilling', as it were. Certainly, there is some evidence of this in the case of young people leaving children's homes (Lupton 1985). There is also evidence from the same source and also from Carlisle's (1996; this volume) study of ex-prisoners that lack of adequate advice and assistance to people leaving institutions such as children's homes and prisons makes it more difficult for them to obtain accommodation. Higate (this volume) offers a tentative explanation of how this process occurs in relation to ex-servicemen.

Table 5.3 Experience of institutions

Type of institution	People in hostels and B&Bs (%)		People sleeping rough (%)	
		(Base)		(Base)
Children's home*	15	(1,268)	24	(499)
Foster parents	10	(1,269)	10	(502)
General hospital (3+ months)*	10	(1,273)	21	(503)
Psychiatric unit*	12	(1,268)	20	(500)
Alcohol unit*	7	(1,271)	17	(503)
Drugs unit	3	(1,274)	4	(502)
Young offender's institution*	9	(1,269)	19	(500)
Prison or remand centre*	24	(1,268)	48	(501)
Armed Forces*	19	(1,277)	29	(506)
Any of the above*	44	(1,280)	69	(507)

Source: Single Homeless People Survey data (1991). Own analysis

Note:

* significant at < 0.01

Whichever explanation is the more important, many single homeless people felt they would need to have some kind of support if they
were to move into their own accommodation. This applied to significantly more people sleeping rough than those staying in hostels and
B&Bs: 52 per cent of the former compared with 59 per cent of the
latter said they would need help of some sort. The help that they felt
was needed included assistance or advice with housekeeping and
money management, medical help, social work support and compan-
ionship. This suggests that homelessness in 1991 was not only a
housing problem but also a social work one.

The above data on support needs combined with the fact that one
in eight people in both samples described themselves as long-term
sick or disabled and the high incidence of health problems among
rough sleepers in particular, suggest that by no means all homeless
single people who could be regarded as 'vulnerable' necessarily get
rehoused by local authorities. Of course, vulnerability is a matter for
local authorities to determine, and they can only do so where they
have received an application by homeless people themselves or have
had a referral made to them. Interestingly, among those who said
they were either long-term sick/disabled or retired, 42 per cent in the
rough-sleeping sample and 21 per cent in the hostel and B&B sam-

ple said they had approached the council as homeless in the previous twelve months. Pleace (this volume) discusses the resettlement of single people who have been accepted for rehousing on the grounds of their vulnerability.

A further aspect of disadvantage which the great majority of single homeless people were experiencing was in relation to the labour market. About nine out of ten people were not in paid employment in the week prior to the survey. About two-fifths of both samples were unemployed and looking for work, and about one in eight described themselves as being long-term unemployed or disabled. However, as Table 5.4 shows, there were some significant differences in employment status between people in hostels and B&Bs and rough sleepers. The main differences were that, in the week before the survey, people sleeping rough were more likely to have been unemployed but not looking for work, while those in hostels and B&Bs were more likely to have been retired or in some other situation such as on a government training scheme or staying in a drug unit.

In most cases single homeless people had not worked for a long time. Only about one in six of the people who were not in paid work during the week prior to the survey had been in employment in the previous six months. A similar proportion had not worked for ten or more years. Just over half of both samples had not worked for at least two years or had never worked.

Table 5.4 Employment status of single homeless people*

	People in hostels and B&Bs (%)	People sleeping rough (%)
In paid work	10	7
Unemployed and looking for work	43	47
Unemployed and not looking for work	13	25
Long-term sick and disabled	13	14
Retired	10	3
Other	10	5
Total	100	100
(Base)	(1271)	(499)

Source: Single Homeless People Survey data (1991). Own analysis
Note:
* significant at < 0.01

The group discussions carried out as part of the research illustrated how being homeless, and particularly sleeping rough, made it so much more difficult for people to get and to hold down paid employment. At the same time they also illustrated how being out of work made it difficult for single homeless people to obtain permanent accommodation (Anderson *et al.* 1993). This again demonstrates the interaction which exists between homelessness and other aspects of disadvantage and discrimination.

Since only a small minority of single homeless people were in paid employment, it is hardly surprising that a disproportionate share of them were dependent upon state benefits of one sort or another – particularly Income Support – to get by (Table 5.5). More hostel and B&B residents were receiving Income Support than people sleeping rough, a difference that may reflect the additional obstacles that rough sleepers may face in claiming benefits from the Benefits Agency (Anderson *et al.* 1993). The most marked difference, however, was that a fifth of rough sleepers, compared with hardly any people in hostels and B&Bs, admitted to begging.

Unlike Income Support, which – once a successful claim has been made – provides a regular flow of income, begging is a precarious source of income and one which can result in prosecution under the

Table 5.5 Income sources and average amounts

	% receiving income from each source		Median amount of income received	
	People in hostels and B&Bs	People sleeping rough	People in hostels and B&Bs	People sleeping rough
			£pw	£pw
Paid work*	11	7	76	60
Unemployment benefit	10	7	40	40
Income support*	56	40	35	39
Other state benefits*	21	16	53	40
Begging*	2	21	10	20
Busking*	1	3	24	23
Other sources	9	7	39	20
All sources	92	80	39	39

Source: Single Homeless People Survey data (1991). Own analysis
Note:
* significant at < 0.01

1824 Vagrancy Act. In 1989, 1,402 people were prosecuted under this legislation (Anderson 1993). Apart from the problem of being arrested or moved on by the police, begging was felt to be a demeaning way of obtaining money by many of the single homeless people who participated in the group discussions. The survey data also suggest that begging is not a particularly remunerative source of income. The median income from this source (in 1991 prices) during the week prior to the survey was £20 among people sleeping rough and £10 among those in hostels and B&B accommodation (Anderson *et al.* 1993).

The median *total* income from all sources in the previous week was £39 for both groups of single homeless people. This works out at less than £6 per day. A minority of respondents – 8 per cent of people in hostels and B&Bs compared with 20 per cent of people who were sleeping rough – said that they had no income at all in the previous week. However, most people sleeping rough and a minority of people in hostels and B&Bs (78 per cent compared with 16 per cent) had received free food, clothing or other help in kind during the previous week. The great majority (89 per cent) of rough sleepers who did not admit to receiving any income in the previous week said they had benefited from free food or other help. This reliance on help in kind reflects the fairly extensive provision of soup runs and day centres in central London, and to a lesser extent elsewhere, when the survey was carried out (Anderson 1993). Soup runs – most of which provided solid meals and tea rather than soup – appeared to be playing a vital role in helping to feed, and by implication to keep alive, many rough sleepers.

THE EXPERIENCE OF SLEEPING ROUGH

By definition, all of the people interviewed in day centres or at soup runs had slept rough at least once during the previous seven days. In addition, and despite the many significant differences between the two samples, 41 per cent of people interviewed in hostels and B&Bs had also slept rough at least once during the previous twelve months. This finding raises at least two important questions about the people in hostels and B&Bs who had slept rough.

First, were they similar to, or different from, either the other people in hostels and B&Bs (who had not slept rough) or the people in the rough-sleeping sample? In fact, they appear to be different from both groups on a range of dimensions, including gender, age, ethnic background, experience of institutions and employment status (Table 5.6).

Compared with people in the rough-sleeping sample, a significantly higher percentage of people in the hostel sample who had experience of sleeping rough in the previous year were women (17 per cent compared with 9 per cent). This difference reflects the fact that a much higher percentage of people in hostels and B&Bs than in the rough sleepers' survey were women. None the less, among people in hostels and B&Bs who had *not* slept rough, the percentage who were women was higher still at 26 per cent. A similar pattern is revealed when ethnic background is examined. Compared with people in the rough-sleeping sample, more people in hostels and B&Bs who had slept rough were from minority (non-White) ethnic groups, although it was not as high as the proportion of people from groups who had not slept rough.

In the case of age, however, the survey reveals that people in hostels and B&Bs who had experience of sleeping rough in the previous year were on average significantly younger than the other people in hostels and B&Bs and also younger than people in the rough-sleeping sample. It appears, therefore, that both younger and older single homeless people are more willing to stay in hostels and B&Bs, or have less need to sleep rough, than their middle-aged counterparts. So far as old people are concerned, the evidence suggests that homeless people find it more difficult to cope with the rigours of sleeping rough when they get old and consequently are more inclined to seek shelter in hostels. Moreover, another reason why there are fewer elderly people sleeping rough than in hostels may be that they die earlier. A study of death certificates in London found that the average age at death of people recorded as having no fixed abode was only 47 years. That is about one third – or, put differently, a quarter of a century – less than the national average life expectancy of 73 for men and 79 for women among the general population (Keyes and Kennedy 1992).

People in hostels and B&Bs who had slept rough in the previous twelve months were significantly more likely to have had experience of being in an institution than other people in hostels and B&Bs, but less likely than people in the rough-sleeping sample. The employment status of people in hostels and B&Bs who had slept rough was also significantly different from that of others in the sample who had not slept rough. The former were much more likely than the latter to have been unemployed and looking for work. In addition, while only 2 per cent of those who had slept rough in the previous twelve

Table 5.6 Characteristics of single homeless people who had had slept rough in the previous 12 months compared with those who had not

	People in hostels and B&Bs who had not slept rough in previous 12 months (%)	People in hostels and B&Bs who had slept rough in previous12 months (%)	People sleeping rough (%)
Gender*			
Female	26	17	9
Male	74	84	91
Age*			
16 to 17	3	10	2
18 to 24	22	35	14
24 to 44	36	38	46
45 to 59	20	14	28
60+	19	3	9
Don't know/can't recall	1	1	1
Ethnic group*			
White	70	83	97
Black & other	30	17	3
Employment status*			
Unemployed & looking for work	44	58	50
Unemployed & not looking for work	14	16	27
Long-term sick & disabled	14	16	15
Retired	15	2	3
Other	13	9	6
Experience of an institution*	39	58	69

Source: Single Homeless People Survey data (1991). Own analysis

Note:
* significant at < 0.01

months were retired, 15 per cent of those who had not slept rough were in this category. Again, however, the employment situation of people in hostels and B&Bs who had slept rough was significantly different from that of people in the rough-sleeping sample. The former were more likely to have been unemployed but looking for work in the week prior to the survey, while the latter were more likely to have been unemployed but not looking for work.

The second question is whether the experience of sleeping rough of people interviewed in hostels and B&Bs was similar to or different from that of the people in the rough-sleeping sample? In fact, the evidence suggests that, comparing the two samples as whole, it was different. People in hostels and B&Bs who had slept rough during the previous twelve months had done so for shorter periods than people in the rough-sleeping sample. Table 5.7 shows the *longest continuous, single period* during which people had slept rough in the previous twelve months. Among people in hostels and B&Bs who had slept rough, 41 per cent had done so for less than a week at most, but this was true for only 8 per cent of people in the rough sleepers' survey. At the other extreme, 50 per cent of people in the rough sleepers' survey, compared with only 14 per cent of those interviewed in

Table 5.7 Longest continuous period, and total time, spent sleeping rough in the previous 12 months

Period	Longest continuous period spent sleeping rough*		Total time spent sleeping rough*	
	People in hostels and B&Bs(%)	People sleeping rough (%)	People in hostels and B&Bs (%)	People sleeping rough (%)
Less than 1 week	41	8	33	4
1 week, less than 1 month	21	13	19	9
1 month, less than 6 months	23	28	26	23
6 months or more	14	50	21	64
Don't know/can't recall	—	1	1	1
Total	100	100	100	100
(Base)	(346)	(461)	(346)	(507)

Source: Single Homeless People Survey data (1991). Own analysis
Note:
* significant at < 0.01

hostels and B&Bs, had slept rough continuously for six months or more during the previous year.

Not only was the longest single incidence of sleeping rough much shorter on average among the people interviewed in hostels and B&Bs who had slept rough in the previous year, but the *total time* they had spent sleeping rough had also been much shorter. As Table 5.7 shows, among people in hostels and B&Bs who had spent time during the previous year sleeping rough, 33 per cent had in total spent less than a week in that way. By contrast, only 4 per cent of those in the rough sleepers' survey had spent less than a week in total sleeping rough. At the other extreme, whereas only 21 per cent of those in hostels and B&Bs who had slept rough during the previous year had spent a total of six months or more doing so, this was true of 64 per cent of people interviewed in the rough sleepers' survey.

For a small minority of those who had slept rough there was a seasonality to their doing so and, perhaps not surprisingly, in the great majority of these cases, they did so in the summer months. The two most commonly cited reasons why people slept rough were that there was no accommodation available or (to a lesser extent) that they could not afford the accommodation that was available. A minority of both samples said that they had problems – such as drug or alcohol dependency – which prevented them from staying in accommodation and hence led them to sleep rough. Very few single homeless people said that they slept rough either because they preferred or liked doing so or because it was a way of life that they had got used to.

CURRENT OR MOST RECENT ACCOMMODATION

Hostels operate a variety of practices in relation both to admission criteria and the maximum permitted length of stay. While some hostels have an open access policy, with few restrictions on who may stay in them, others confine admission to particular groups of homeless people, such as young adults and women. Likewise, some hostels allow residents to stay for unlimited periods of time while others seek to restrict length of stays to a definite period (Garside *et al.* 1990; Neale 1996). There is some evidence that in London the lack of move-on accommodation for residents had caused hostels to 'silt up', with the result that maximum lengths of stay have had to be reassessed and extended in some cases (Spaull and Rowe 1992).

Nevertheless, hostels and B&Bs provide a very insecure form of accommodation and one that is designed to be only temporary in

Table 5.8 Length of stay in present or most recent accommodation

Length of stay	People in hostels and B&Bs (current accommodation)(%)	People sleeping rough (most recent accommodation)(%)
Less than 1 week	7	31
1 week, less than 1 month	14	18
1 month, less than 6 months	33	27
6 months, less than 1 year	14	7
1+ years	33	15
Don't know/can't recall	1	2
Total	100	100
(Base)	(1,266)	(262)

Source: Single Homeless People Survey data (1991). Own analysis
Note:
* significant at < 0.01

duration. As Table 5.8 shows, 20 per cent had been resident for less than a month. At the other extreme, 33 per cent had been living in their current accommodation for one or more years. In fact, 11 per cent had been there for five or more years. Thus it appears that hostels and B&Bs cater for a dual market among the single homeless: while some residents stay for quite short periods, many others live there for extended periods, making it more like permanent than temporary accommodation. Indeed, 13 per cent of hostel and B&B residents described the accommodation as their home (Anderson *et al.* 1993).

Just as some people interviewed in hostels and B&Bs had spent time sleeping rough during the previous twelve months, so too some people interviewed at day centres or soup runs had stayed in accommodation. Indeed, one in six people in the rough sleepers' sample had spent the night prior to the survey in accommodation, though all had slept rough at least once during the previous week. Among those who had slept rough in the night before the survey, three out of ten had last stayed in accommodation during the previous month, while a third had not done so for a year or more. Thus, a substantial minority of people could be regarded as long-term or chronic rough sleepers.

Altogether, two-thirds of people in the rough-sleeping sample had stayed in some form of accommodation during the previous year. However, the period during which they had occupied accommodation in their most recent stay was in most cases quite short. Almost a half of people in the rough-sleeping sample had stayed for less than a month in their most recent accommodation, while only one in seven had been resident for a year or more.

Among people sleeping rough who had spent at least one night in accommodation in the previous twelve months, 16 per cent had last lived in their own house, flat or bedsit. Thus only a minority had moved straight from their own home into sleeping rough. In fact, the most common (46 per cent) type of place that people in the rough-sleeping sample had stayed in last was a hostel, night shelter or B&B hotel. Only 4 per cent had last stayed in accommodation that belonged to their parents (or foster parents). A further 17 per cent had last stayed in accommodation belonging to a friend or relative before (their present episode of) sleeping rough. Another 7 per cent had last stayed in a squat, an inherently insecure form of accommodation. Finally, 6 per cent had been in an institution of some sort – such as a children's home, prison, psychiatric unit, drug or alcohol unit, or general hospital – in their most recent stay in accommodation. In other words, they had moved directly from staying in an institution to living on the streets.

CONCLUSIONS

Perhaps the most striking finding from the 1991 survey is the very diverse characteristics of single people who were homeless (Anderson 1994; Deacon et al. 1995). This heterogeneity (cf. Drake et al. 1982) is not well captured in the rather simple stereotypes that have often pervaded presentations of such people in the mass media and in political debates. Moreover, the apparent causes of their homelessness are also very diverse, as the report of the survey makes clear (Anderson et al. 1993).

Nevertheless, what this chapter has demonstrated is that there were many statistically significant differences between the characteristics of single homeless people staying in hostels, night shelters and B&B hotels and those who were currently sleeping rough. In addition, within the group of people staying in hostels, there were many significant differences between those who had slept rough on at least one occasion in the previous twelve months and those who had not done so. Likewise, there were significant differences between people in hostels who had slept rough in the previous twelve months and people who were currently sleeping rough.

Thus, some single homeless people were long-term residents of hostels and had no recent experience of sleeping rough. Others were long-term rough sleepers who had little or no experience of staying in hostels or other forms of temporary accommodation. Yet others were staying in hostels but had experienced more or less lengthy periods of sleeping rough in the previous year. And of course some single homeless people were either staying in hostels and B&Bs or sleeping rough for the first time since becoming homeless (cf. Randall and Brown 1996).

Comparing the people who were staying in hostels and B&Bs in 1991 with the 1972 survey of hostels and common lodging houses carried out by Digby (1976), it is apparent that there had been some major changes in the characteristics of single homeless people over this period. In particular, there has been a major increase in the share of homelessness accounted for by women, young people, and (probably) Black people. These three trends are not unrelated, since a disproportionate share of homeless people in 1991 were young Black women. Indeed, the treble discrimination and disadvantage which they faced (that is, being under 25, female and Black) seems likely to have increased greatly their probability of being homeless compared with the general population.

It is also clear from the survey results that single homeless people in 1991 suffered from a range of other forms of disadvantage and discrimination. The majority of single homeless people were long-term unemployed, endured worse health than the population at large, had more experience of life in children's homes and penal institutions, and suffered from a high incidence of alcohol and illicit drug dependency. In some of these aspects – such as health and employment status – a question mark exists about which was cause and which was effect (cf. Drake *et al.* 1982). Nevertheless, even where the problem was a consequence rather than a cause, being homeless made it worse. For example, while being long-term unemployed may have made single people more likely to lose their home, once they were homeless it was that much more difficult for them to find and hold down a job.

It is also apparent from the survey results that, even if they were to have obtained a house or flat of their own, many single homeless people would have required community care or other forms of assistance and advice to maintain the tenancy of it. Whether or not these needs preceded their homelessness or were among the factors behind it is not clear and indeed may well have varied between individuals.

At any rate, the incidence of these needs is higher than that found in the 1978 survey of Drake *et al.* (though comparisons with that study are not straightforward). Single homelessness in 1991 was not just about a lack of housing, but was also a community care problem. Indeed, the group discussions suggested that the experience of homelessness itself – particularly that of spending extended periods sleeping rough – made it difficult for people to get by in their own accommodation. In consequence, the two facets of homelessness – lack of housing and difficulty in maintaining an independent home – are best regarded as intertwined rather than separate problems. In this respect at least, the emphasis on outreach and resettlement work together with the provision of temporary and permanent accommodation that characterises the Rough Sleepers Initiative (Randall and Brown 1996) seems to be a good starting point for tackling the problem of rough sleeping.

NOTE

1 Thanks are due to Isobel Anderson and Deborah Quilgars, who worked with me on the 1991 survey of single homeless people and to the Department of the Environment for funding it. Responsibility for the re-analysis of the data and for the arguments set out in this chapter rests with the author.

Chapter 6

Mortgage arrears, mortgage possessions and homelessness

Janet Ford

HOMELESSNESS AND OWNER OCCUPATION

Until the early 1980s, there was an assumption that once households had gained access to owner occupation their future as owners was unproblematic. There was a view, widely held by individuals and many commentators, that buying a house was one of the best investments available, with house-price inflation and rising incomes providing a cushion against the unlikely event of any financial difficulties. Thus there was little association between owner occupation and homelessness, save with respect to issues of relationship breakdown, where a number of studies pointed to the risk of homelessness amongst those who left the matrimonial home (Tunnard 1976; Sullivan 1986).

During the 1980s, however, an association between homelessness and owner occupation became clearer, signified by the rise in the number of households losing their property as a result of mortgage arrears and so possession of their property. In 1981, 4,870 households lost their homes in this manner. By 1987, the figure was 26,390 and in 1991, the numbers peaked at 75,540.

The figures on those losing their property cited above can, however, be compared with another set of figures that suggest that the scale of homelessness resulting from mortgage possession is much smaller. In 1987, only 9 per cent of those officially designated as homeless in England were so as a result of mortgage arrears, approximately 10,120 (of the total of 26,390) households in possession. The percentage figure then fell but by 1991 had risen again to 12 per cent of all acceptances (18,000). By 1993, the figure had fallen to eight per cent, and it appears to have stabilised at this level with the figure for 1995 also being 8 per cent.

The 'gap' between these two sets of figures comes about because the majority of mortgagors who lose their property through possession either have no eligibility for rehousing as officially homeless, or, if they are eligible, choose not to approach the local authority (Ford *et al.* 1995). Any ineligibility results from potential applicants not qualifying as being 'in priority need' under the homelessness legislation (typically because they are households without children), or because the possession process was a voluntary as opposed to a compulsory one. Voluntary possession, which has been running at between 30 and 40 per cent of possessions per annum, entails households returning the property to the lender (for example, either by abandoning it or posting back the keys) as opposed to losing their property as a result of a judicial process and court order for possession. Where possession is voluntary, local authorities have the possibility of deeming the homelessness *intentional*, and so outside their legislative responsibilities. Why households may take this course of action is discussed elsewhere (Ford 1993, 1995).

Table 6.1 draws some of the measures of homelessness together and shows that no more than 30 per cent of all households in possession (that is, both voluntary and compulsory possession) and no more than 50 per cent of those obtained with a court order (compulsory possessions) are accepted by the local authority as homeless. A substantial proportion of households, homeless because of mortgage possession, are simply not *officially recognised* as such, and the term the 'unrecognised' homeless is used in this chapter to refer to these people. Table 6.1 also shows that the percentage of those in possession, and rehoused following acceptance as officially homeless, has been falling and in 1993 constituted less than a fifth of all possession cases. Thus, reliance on the local authority acceptances as a measure of homelessness resulting from mortgage arrears grossly understates the extent of the problem.

Possession is a consequence of financial difficulties and mortgage arrears. However, the number of possessions does not necessarily reflect the number of borrowers in serious arrears. Prior to 1991, practically all borrowers with long-term arrears were taken into possession. During 1991, this relationship changed and the number in long-term arrears began to outstrip the number taken into possession. This relationship has continued, so that in 1995, there were roughly 50,000 possessions, but more than 85,000 borrowers with arrears of twelve or more months. Equally, not all borrowers summonsed in the court for possession proceedings are taken into possession.

Table 6.1 Mortgage possessions and local authority acceptances for homelessness, England

	1990	1991	1992	1993	1994	1995
Total LA homelessness acceptances	145,800	151,720	148,980	137,980	127,290	125,640
Percentage LA acceptances	9	12	10	8	8	8
due to mortgage arrears	13,122	18,206	14,825	11,038	10,183	10,051
CML figures for no. of possessions						
(a) all possessions	43,890	75,540	68,540	58,540	49,190	49,410
(b) by court order*	26,334	45,324	41,124	35,124	32,957	32,610
Percentage of possession cases rehoused by LA						
(a) of all possessions	30	24	22	19	21	20
(b) of compulsory possessions	50	40	36	32	31	31

Sources: Wilcox, S. (1996) *Housing Review 1996/97*, York: Joseph Rowntree Foundation and Ford, J. (1994) *Problematic Home Ownership*, Loughborough: Loughborough University and Joseph Rowntree Foundation. Own analysis
Notes:
* In the early 1990s approximately 40% of possessions were voluntary

The trends identified above suggest that the relationships between arrears, possessions, official and unrecognised homelessness are complex and that trends on one measure cannot necessarily be read off directly from the others. This chapter aims to address some of the issues surrounding these relationships and in particular it will consider four issues. First, how can we account for the growth of mortgage arrears and possessions and consequent homelessness in the late 1980s and early 1990s? Second, the chapter will examine the process of becoming homeless, focusing primarily on a consideration of the compulsory possession process. Third, it will take up the question of the rehousing of the unrecognised homeless, and finally, briefly consider the likely future extent of possessions and associated homelessness and some outstanding policy issues.

THE GROWTH OF MORTGAGE ARREARS AND POSSESSIONS

To a greater or lesser extent, the expansion of owner occupation has been a policy objective of all post-war governments in Britain. By fits and starts, home ownership grew from a minority tenure at the start of the Second World War to a position in 1996 where 67 per cent of all households, over 14 million, are now owners; more than 10.5 million of them buying their home with a mortgage. The expansion reflects the stated aspirations of consumers who, as real incomes grew, increasingly had the means to buy; the profit aspirations of the property and finance sectors of the economy; and, particularly in the 1980s, the strength of ideological influences in favour of depoliticising welfare, emphasising individual responsibility and constraining local authority activity.

The concerns of this chapter do not require any further historical account of the growth of owner occupation – for further development, see Malpass and Murie (1994) and Boddy (1980). Rather, the focus needs to be placed on the most recent expansion which spanned the 1980s and on the ways in which housing policy, together with fiscal and wider economic measures, came together first to facilitate the expansion of households' access to home ownership, and then to jeopardise households' ability to maintain their financial commitments. Thus, the understanding of the rise of arrears, possessions and the associated homelessness is closely connected to issues of policy and the operation of the housing market.

The 1980s expansion of owner occupation

Two areas of government policy helped fuel the 1980s growth in owner occupation: the introduction of the 'Right to Buy' in the 1980 Housing Act in the context of a restriction on new house building by local authorities; and the deregulation of credit markets achieved through the 1985 Financial Services Act and 1986 Building Societies Act. The 1980 Housing Act allowed existing tenants to purchase their properties at a discount and with a right to a mortgage (Forrest and Murie 1988). The 1985 and 1986 Acts ended credit rationing and created an enlarged and highly competitive credit market. Unconstrained credit and competition to lend resulted in some relaxation of lending criteria and a rapid rise in the number of mortgage advances to first-time buyers. The number of first-time buyers grew from 318,000 in 1981 to 619,000 in 1986. A substantial proportion of new buyers were lower income households (DSS 1992). As a proportion of all home-buying households, those in the bottom income decile grew from 11 per cent to 27 per cent (before housing costs) between 1979 and 1990/91. This was a result of an increase in pensioner and economically inactive mortgagors, but also a growth in the percentage of mortgagors in full-time employment. Over the same period, amongst skilled manual workers, home ownership grew from 32 to 59 per cent and from 9 per cent each of semi- and unskilled workers to 42 per cent and 25 per cent respectively.

The impact of rising demand, however, reinforced already existing tendencies towards house-price inflation, and as house prices rose strongly, those outside the market were encouraged to enter, often concerned that any further delay might price them out of the market. Demand was therefore boosted still further. An additional impetus to entry (and so house-price inflation) came in 1988 when the Chancellor of the Exchequer gave three months' notice of his intention to end the practice of allowing double tax relief on mortgage interest (MIRAS) where two (unrelated) people purchased together.

The cost impact of the changes sketched out above can be seen in Table 6.2. A comparison of 1980, 1985 and 1990 shows that on every measure the average costs associated with home ownership increased. The final column indicates the position in 1995/96, and discussion of the current situation will be picked up towards the end of the chapter.

Table 6.2 Changes in the financial characteristics of mortgages,
United Kingdom, 1980, 1985, 1990, 1995

	1980	*1985*	*1990*	*1995*
Average house prices (1990 = 100)	35	50	100	93
Average advance as % of house price (ftb)	73.8	85.3	82.5	89.0
Average advance as % of house price (foo)	46.1	59.2	59.3	64.2
Average advance to average income (ftb)	1.67	1.94	2.19	2.21
Average advance to average income (foo)	1.54	1.83	2.00	1.99
Average repayment as % of average income (ftb)	19.0	20.0	28.1	18.9
Average repayment as % of average income (foo)	17.5	19.0	24.6	16.6
Mortgage interest rates	14.9	13.2	15.0	7.0

Source: Wilcox, S. (1996) *Housing Review 1996/97*, York: Joseph Rowntree
Foundation. Own analysis
Notes:
ftb = first-time buyer
foo = former owner occupier

Recessionary pressures

By the late 1980s, the pressures generated in the housing market by the
policy agenda were accentuating wider economic difficulties, in particular inflation, amplifying the routine cyclical processes in the economy and housing market to the status of 'boom and bust' (Maclennan
1994). The government, faced with rising inflation, sought to control
it through the interest-rate mechanism and hence mortgage interest
rates rose. Whereas they had been 9.5 per cent in May 1988, by February 1990 they were 15.4 per cent, contributing to the increase in
average United Kingdom weekly mortgage repayments, which rose
from almost £38 a week to over £60 (Murphy 1994). The position was
particularly acute for two sets of borrowers: those who had bought
towards or at the height of the boom with high loan-to-value and loan-
to-income ratios; and borrowers whose access had been secured by
the use of low-start, discounted mortgages or fixed-rate/fixed-duration
mortgages which happened to end as interest rates rose. Sometimes
these two sets of circumstances overlapped.

Within the economy generally, rising interest rates slowed consumer demand and in 1990 the rate of unemployment began to

increase, peaking at 10.6 per cent in January 1993. Like previous recessions, manual and unskilled workers were vulnerable to unemployment (and many more of them were home owners in 1990 than had been in 1980), but in contrast to previous recessions, so were professional and managerial workers (Hogarth *et al.* 1996). The recession also impacted initially and heavily in the South of England (where house-price rises and levels of borrowing had been highest), only later rippling out to the Midlands and the North.

As interest rates and unemployment rose, the impact on the housing market was first stagnation and then a severe depression. The number of transactions fell, as did the number of mortgage advances and also house prices (Forrest and Murie 1994), although these developments had a varied geographical impact. The phenomenon of negative equity emerged where people owed more than the market value of their property (Dorling and Cornford 1995; Forrest *et al.* 1994). This reduced sales yet further and reinforced the downward pressures in the housing market.

The recessionary forces, in the context of the previous housing boom – easy access to credit and more highly geared borrowers – created a substantial number of financial problems for mortgagors and the available statistics began to record increases in both arrears and possessions. Table 6.3 below, drawn from lenders' records, shows that the number of households owing three or more monthly payments rose from 202,600 in 1989 to a peak in excess of 580,000 in 1991. By 1993 the figure had barely changed (558,400). Properties taken into possession rose in the mid-1980s, then fell, but rose again from 15,810 in 1989 to a peak of 75,540 in 1991. Since then, possessions have fallen, but have levelled out at around 50,000 per year (CML 1996). As noted above, before 1991, long-term arrears were 'managed' by lenders and/or borrowers through forced or voluntary sales. That position changed in 1991. The number of possessions no longer matches the number with longer-term arrears, and the pool of long-term arrears (over six months' missed payments) is still close to 200,000 households. These are potentially homeless individuals and families.

The statistics above, although useful, are nevertheless limited, and there is a well-developed critique of the statistics on arrears and possessions (Doling *et al.* 1989; Ford 1993; Ford *et al.* 1995). Recent survey work has overcome a number of the problems, in particular the reliance on lenders for data and the emphasis on the stock of arrears rather than their incidence (Ford *et al.* 1995; Green *et al.*

Table 6.3 Mortgage arrears and possessions, 1985–96

	1980	1985	1987	1989	1991	1993	1995
Number of mortgages at year end (000s)	6,210	7,717	8,283	9,125	9,185	10,137	10,510
Repossessions during year	3,480	19,300	26,390	15,810	75,540	58,540	49,410
Cases in mortgage arrears							
12+ months' arrears	—	13,120	14,960	13,840	91,740	151,810	85,200
6–12 months' arrears	15,530	57,110	55,490	66,800	183,610	164,620	126,670
3–5 months' arrears	—	97,000	121,000	122,000	305,500	242,050	179,050
2 months' arrears	—	140,000	164,400	153,900	269,800	198,400	119,715

Sources: Council of Mortgage Lenders, Housing Finance data and Ford, J. (1980–96) data collected for *Roof* (figures for 2 and 3–5 months' arrears). Own analysis

Notes:
Properties taken into posession include those voluntarily surrendered. Figures for 6–12 and 12+ months' arrears are for the end of the year. 2 and 3–5 months' arrears figures are for the March of the year. Changes in the mortgage rate have the effect of changing monthly repayments and hence the number of months in arrears which a given amount represents

1996). These recent surveys show the extent to which mortgagors face financial difficulties with their mortgages but manage to pay, as well as the variety of missed payment patterns that contribute to the arrears figures. They also provide information on the incidence as well as the stock of arrears at any one time. Using the period 1991–94, Ford *et al.* (1995) showed that roughly one in five home buyers had been 'at risk' (either in terms of financial difficulties or missed payments). Their payment careers were as follows:

- 3 per cent had no current arrears but had previous arrears;
- 3 per cent were having difficulties paying and had arrears previously;
- 1 per cent were in arrears again, having cleared previous arrears;
- 1 per cent had been in arrears for the whole of the period under consideration;
- 3 per cent had fallen into arrears for the first time in the last three years;
- 9 per cent had no arrears over the period but had current payment difficulties.

A range of social and economic policies in the 1980s and 1990s have therefore raised the risks faced by mortgagors and arrears have risen. Although they are now below their peak, they remain substantial. In 1996, around one in every twenty home-buying households missed at least two months' mortgage payments. However, not everyone in arrears finds themselves giving possession, and the relationship between arrears and possessions is a variable one. Even so, since the start of 1991, in excess of 300,000 households have lost their property in this manner. The next section focuses on some key processes that contribute to the rate at which arrears are 'converted' to possessions and result in homeless households.

BECOMING HOMELESS

Many more people are at risk of homelessness from arrears and possession than ever become homeless. There are a number of factors that contribute to any understanding of the ways in which arrears link to possessions; these include the capacity of those in default to repay, lender forbearance, borrowers' attitudes and decisions, government intervention, the nature of the both public and private safety net systems and the nature of the judicial possession process. Research shows, for example, that around one in six of those owing at least three months' payments manage to meet their normal monthly payment and gradually repay their arrears (Ford *et al.* 1995). The ability to repay depends on a range of factors, including the households' financial circumstances, their commitment to remaining owners and the terms and conditions of repayment set by lenders. The nature of lenders' forbearance is also a contributory factor, and research shows that there is a range of decisions taken by lenders as to how they will manage arrears. Both Ford *et al.* (1995) and NACAB (1995) have noted that some lenders will accept interest-only payments, or substantially reduced payments for (varying) periods of time, whereas others will not and proceed to a court summons for possession much more rapidly. There is an important question, but not one pursued here, as to whether forbearance strategies help people repay, or merely delay possession, but it is likely that both these outcomes will occur.

A number of borrowers in arrears have also had some protection from possession afforded to them as a result of a government intervention in December 1991. At that time, and as a result of the growing public and political concern about rising possessions, lenders and the government entered into an agreement whereby lenders would not possess borrowers on Income Support and in receipt of mortgage interest payments (ISMI). In return, the government instituted the payment of such mortgage interest directly from the Department of Social Security to lenders – see Ford and Wilcox (1992) and Ford *et al.* (1995) for a full discussion of these developments. Lenders have varied in the extent to which they have interpreted the agreement as referring only to borrowers in receipt of 100 per cent ISMI or have been willing to desist from seeking possession where the eligible interest is less than 100 per cent. The outcome has been a prevention of possession, and so homelessness, perhaps in the order of around 10,000 households. The agreement has though been in part responsible for the continuing high level of long-term arrears. Amongst some lenders, more than 50 per cent of borrowers with long-term arrears are ISMI claimants.

However, the likelihood of possession may well increase once judicial proceedings are instituted, and the rest of this section explores the nature of this key process in more detail. The possession process plays two roles with respect to homelessness. First, it is a clear route to homelessness, as a possession order, if executed, reclaims the property for the lender, if necessary by the bailiffs evicting the occupants. Evidence of possession via a court order is also a necessary, if not sufficient, requirement of acceptance by the local authority as officially homeless. Second, the possession process may afford protection from homelessness by giving the borrower a further opportunity to repay. Thus, not everyone who is summonsed in court for possession necessarily ends up losing their property. In 1995, for example, there were 84,170 actions entered for mortgage possession (LCD 1996), but only around 32,000 cases where possession via a court order was the end result (CML 1996). Other actions entered were either dismissed, adjourned or granted a suspended order, allowing repayment of the arrears over time. The outcome of the possession process is highly contingent, dependent on the judicial framework, the circumstances of borrowers and the attitudes of lenders (plaintiffs), borrowers (defendants) and district judges. Surrounding and informing these aspects are wider public and political attitudes to housing policy and the expansion of home ownership in particular.

Borrowers in arrears are in breach of their mortgage contract with the lender and creditors have right of redress, typically through the county courts under the 1970 Administration of Justice Act. Once arrears total at least two months' payments, borrowers can be summonsed for possession and given a date for a hearing in the county courts. Unlike enforcement for most other debts, cases are no longer heard in open court but privately 'in chambers', where both defendant and plaintiff have the right of representation. The enforcement process has administrative and judicial rules and preferred procedures; for example, lenders must provide sworn affidavits, while defendants are encouraged to submit relevant information to the court, but cannot be denied a hearing in its absence. Centrally, however, the district judge has discretion as to the outcome of the hearing; in particular, whether a case is dismissed, adjourned, granted an outright order for possession or a suspended order, and the terms and conditions that attach to the latter. Here, a key issue is the decision the judge makes as to what length of time the borrower can have to repay the arrears, known as the 'reasonable period'.

Analysis of court records relating to mortgage possession shows that the balance of outcomes has varied over time, indicating some change in the nature of the discretionary decisions made. In particular, in the early 1990s, the ratio of outright orders to suspended orders fell (LCD 1991, 1996). The time people were given to repay their arrears also lengthened. By 1993–94, the average length of the reasonable period was between three and a half and four years (Ford *et al.* 1995), whereas in the mid-1980s it had been much shorter (Doling *et al.* 1984). Other studies have also indicated shifts in the assessment of cases by district judges in the 1990s. Griffith (1993), observing cases in one county court, noted how over a period of two years, one judge moved from first determining the reasonable period as between twelve and eighteen months, to a longer period in order 'to see whether the defendant and [her] family can retain a roof above their heads which they've striven [for] so long'. He then began granting suspended orders that required only the repayment of the normal monthly payments, with consideration of the arrears either adjourned to a later date or 'held over in the hope that the recession will recede and the [defendant] will be able to find work and pay'.

In terms of the development of a homeless career, by the early 1990s, a greater proportion of borrowers found that the court process offered a way to slow, or even prevent their entry into homelessness. But a key question is why these changes came about. The explanation explored here involves recognising the ways in which the judicial enforcement process, including the discretionary decisions of judges, is a social process, structured and informed by societal views and concerns on the one hand and the behaviour of defendants on the other. Thus homelessness too must be seen as reflecting and so influenced by these processes.

Viewing enforcement as a social process owes much to the work of Rock (1973) and Cain (1986). Neither writer was specifically concerned with mortgage default – when Rock did his research it was practically non-existent – but their perspectives remain pertinent, and account well for the continuities and changes in the processes and outcomes associated with mortgage possession. Both writers, to varying degrees, characterised enforcement as a process with low visibility, poorly understood by defendants, involved in processing people via a stream of 'ever more threatening actions' but which nevertheless could be reversed at any point by payment. Court officials classified defendants by their actions, which signified both attitude and motivation, and provided the rationale for subsequent decisions. Both Rock and Cain viewed enforcement as lacking external scrutiny (because of public unawareness and the lack of any politicisation of debt as a social issue), and as a process designed to retain the issue as a private, contractual matter rather than an issue of public concern. Both writers accepted the legitimacy of a process that provides creditors with redress and thereby confidence in their ability to maintain and extend the credit system. Cain, drawing her analysis from traditions within the sociologies of work and occupation, stressed the ways in which registrars (district judges) perceived their role as one of establishing 'fair play'. However, despite this, the presumption of defendant liability necessitated the presentation of a defence. Fair play was brought about through the application of discretion.

These perspectives on enforcement continue to encapsulate much of the nature of the current possession process. In some critical ways, however, the process has been subject to change as the social context and understanding of default has changed, and these in turn have influenced attitudes towards, beliefs about and responses to defaulters. Several factors have contributed to these changes: centrally, the growing public awareness of debt, the growing external scrutiny and politicisation of debt; and the opportunities provided by on-going legal debate.

Changing public awareness

Public awareness of debt, and particularly mortgage default, has increased, potentially challenging the well-routed, blameworthy stereotypes of debtors. In 1973, Rock reported the dearth of public knowledge of default. Although statistics on default are virtually non-existent for the 1970s, the restricted availability of 'mainstream' credit (from banks, building societies, retailers and finance houses) makes it unlikely that many people were themselves in any kind of default or knew others in that position. By contrast, the number of households with any kind of debt stood at 2.3 million in 1992, amongst whom 560,000 had two or more problem debts (Berthoud and Kempson 1992). Specifically with respect to mortgages, and based on a survey in three towns, Maclennan (1994) indicated that a majority of people knew someone currently in mortgage arrears or who had lost their home through possession.

Awareness of mortgage default and its implications also increased through the actions of the media. Since 1988, a continuous stream of articles, and radio and television programmes has highlighted easy access to credit, 'irresponsible' lending, additional borrowing (not often reported as 'irresponsible borrowing' of which there was undoubtedly some), unsympathetic lenders, tough courts and evicted households. These reports were frequently contextualised as affecting borrowers who had acted in good faith, believing and responding to government ideology and policy by, as they often put it, 'standing on their own two feet' but who felt they had subsequently been 'let down' (Ford 1993, 1994). Public interpretations increasingly moved away from seeing debtors as feckless and irresponsible towards a view of them as caught by circumstances beyond their control. Comparing the public statements of even the mid-1980s with those of the early 1990s, the change of emphasis is marked.

Mortgage default also became more directly politicised, most clearly at the end of 1991 when demands by the press and Opposition for government intervention to stem the repossessions crisis led to what became known as the 'mortgage rescue' package as discussed earlier (Ford and Wilcox 1992; Foster 1992; Wilcox and Williams 1996, Ford *et al.* 1995).

The courts, and therefore district judges, were, in one sense at the forefront of changing public awareness. In 1990, the courts faced an increase of almost 60 per cent in the actions entered for possession by mortgagees, from 91,309 to 145,350. There was a further rise to 186,649 in 1991 (LCD 1991). Although the increases were not uniform across the country, few courts were unaffected by them. Extra hearing days were necessary and cases had to be processed more quickly at any one sitting (Nixon and Hunter 1996). District judges could not help being aware of the scale of the emerging problem and its likely causes.

Ford *et al.* (1995) report that a number of judges expressed reservations about the policy that had deregulated the credit market and encouraged over-zealous marketing by some lenders (in particular a number of secondary lenders), the excessive demands for repayment from some lenders, and the high, yet unaccountable level of costs that borrowers had to meet in connection with litigation (Ford *et al.* 1995). Thus, the judges' pursuit of 'fair play' was increasingly in the context of recognising that the issue was less one of borrower fecklessness and more one of borrowers trapped by structural changes and circumstances they could not have predicted, the effects of which they could not control, and where they might need to be afforded some protection. The shift to understanding the issue as more structural than individual can be seen in the 1991 comments of Lord Justice Dillon: 'claims for possession by mortgagees against borrowers who have become unemployed and so unable to keep up the payments under their mortgages have become very common and constitute a serious *social problem'* (author's emphasis) (Dillon 1991).

Some judges were also closely attuned to the political debate and particularly to the 1991 ISMI agreement (see above) which they used to 'protect' some borrowers (Ford *et al.*1995). In one court, the first question asked by the judge to the plaintiff's representative seeking outright possession for a claimant was: 'Are your clients not members of the Council of Mortgage Lenders?' If the answer was 'yes' he continued: 'Did the Council not give an undertaking to the Government not to enforce possession orders against debtors on Income Support in consideration of the payment of benefit to the lender?'

A second influence on the changing outcomes for defendants is the greater awareness of the judicial process and more effective response to it on the part of defendants. From the mid-1980s onwards researchers and campaigning organisations recognised that one of the ways in which defendants might improve their chances of avoiding possessions was to make written representations to, or attend personally at court.

District judges are most easily able to consider exercising discretion in favour of the borrower (usually to award a suspended order for possession), where the borrower attends the hearing. The defendant's position is likely to be strengthened still further where they are well prepared, able to present to the court both an explanation of their current circumstances (the 'defence'), an account of any discussions with their lender and a proposal for recovery. Organisations such as Housing Advice Centres and Citizens' Advice Bureaux have been active in informing borrowers about this, undertaking income and expenditure assessments with defaulters in order to arrive at a sustainable recovery offer (or a recognition that the property cannot be retained) and, where requested, in providing support at the court hearing. Attendance at court by defendants in mortgage possession actions has risen substantially since the mid-1980s and now exceeds 50 per cent of all defendants. A further development, and one increasingly welcomed by court staff, is the establishment of court-based advice services, often, but not always a local advice agency presence (Nixon *et al.* 1996). There are now in excess of sixty courts with such provision and evidence shows that district judges will refer defendants to the service and in some cases rely entirely on the adviser's assessment of a case in deciding the outcome.

For district judges who wish to exercise discretion as expansively as possible, a further influence may well have been the debate stemming from the suggestion that the reasonable period might be interpreted as the lifetime of the mortgage – for a fuller account and analysis of the legal discussion, see Luba *et al.* (1993). This interpretation was first made in the 1970s but the ideas have become more prominent recently, where a case heard on appeal (*Norgan* v.

Cheltenham and Gloucester Building Society, December 1995)
reiterated the view that the court should begin its deliberations with
the presumption that the remaining term of the mortgage was the
reasonable period. Campaigning organisations have made much of
this possibility (NCC 1992; NACAB 1995), but potentially, district
judges may too have come to some reassessment of the term, in the
context of judicial debate.

The argument offered here, that the courts have contributed to a
reduction in the risk of possession (and so homelessness) both
reflecting and responding to changing social, political and legal
processes can, however, be challenged. In particular, some writers
(Stewart, 1996; Nixon and Hunter 1996) have suggested that the role
of the courts in safeguarding the interests of capital (in this instance,
mortgage lenders) remains paramount. In contrast to an analysis that
sees the judiciary as sometimes (but increasingly) redressing the balance of power from lender to borrower, the outcomes of the possession process are viewed as reflecting lenders' economic interests.
Thus the growth in suspended orders noted earlier reflects lenders'
interests in the light of the state of the housing market and the downward economic pressures associated with large numbers of often
poor-quality houses coming onto an already depressed market. This
argument remains to be explored in detail, but will need to address a
number of issues: for example, the extent to which district judges
override the expressed wishes of lenders (of which there is some evidence). This argument also leads to the hypothesis that an upturn in
market conditions will increase the number of possessions as sales
and price movements act to minimise losses to lenders, and this too
will need to be explored.

Housing policy, economic policy and market mechanisms have
been increasingly implicated in the analysis of mortgage default and
possession and, by extension, in the increase in homelessness. This
changing context of attitudes, beliefs, perceptions and externally
generated demands has had consequences for both lay and judicial
views on defendants' liability, on what constitutes 'fair play', and has
encouraged some modification in the previously held processes for
the classification of and responses to defaulters. One outcome has
been a reduction in the extent of homelessness that might otherwise
have resulted.

In proportional terms, the possession process is less of a route to
homelessness now than was previously the case. A lower proportion
of those with arrears enter the judicial process and there is a greater

chance than previously that they will be awarded a suspended order. At best this will prevent possession and homelessness and at worst give the borrower one more chance to see if they can repay, before finally losing their home. There is little available evidence of the extent to which those granted a suspended order do repay and so the extent to which the 'hopes' embodied in a suspended order are realised, but such evidence as there is (Ford 1994) suggests that three out of every five borrowers with a suspended order fail to repay.

Before exploring how those households which lose their owner-occupied homes are rehoused, it is useful to consider briefly who becomes homeless and why. This issue is discussed more fully in Ford *et al.* (1995) and Green *et al.* (1996), but households where the mortgagor(s) is or are unemployed are at greater risk of possession than those in employment, as are self-employed borrowers. Given the gradient of unemployment by socio-economic group, the expansion of owner occupation through its promotion amongst manual workers has clearly increased the sectors vulnerability to arrears and possessions. However, this alone is too simple an explanation, and certainly in the period 1990–94 one in four possessions were amongst professional, managerial and associated workers. In part, this reflects the nature of the early 1990s recession which was both a blue- and white-collar recession, but also the nature of the preceding boom in the housing market as discussed earlier. The pattern was rather different from the one seen in the early 1980s when, despite fewer low-income mortgagors, they were the group that bore the brunt of arrears and possessions, as they bore the brunt of unemployment.

HOUSING THE UNRECOGNISED HOMELESS

Earlier in this chapter, a contrast was drawn between the number of households giving possession in any one year and the number of households rehoused by the local authority following possession. Table 6.1 suggests that a majority of households, homeless as a result of mortgage arrears, are rehoused outside the local authority sector. The ways in which this group of homeless people find housing and the kind of housing they secure is considered briefly below.

'Homelessness' amongst those giving possession may not manifest itself as 'rooflessness'. In large part this is due to the fact that once a possession order is granted there is typically a lapse of twenty-eight days before it is implemented. Those approaching the local authority seeking to be housed as a result of their impending homelessness frequently do so once the possession order is granted. Those who are successful in their application may even move into new (but often temporary) accommodation ahead of eviction. Others who are either deemed ineligible or who do not approach the local authority may also use the period prior to eviction to find somewhere to live, but it is often temporary and/or unsuitable accommodation. The term 'homeless' is therefore still appropriate for households losing their home through possession; most are not initially rehoused in suitable or permanent accommodation and they may remain insecure and mobile for several months.

Households losing their property often have to resort initially to some form of temporary accommodation, only later finding or being allocated something more permanent. This is the case for both the official and unrecognised homeless. Table 6.4 presents data from a sample survey of borrowers taken into possession in England between 1991 and 1994, indicating their initial post-possession housing and the housing they were living in at the point they were interviewed (referred to as the 'final destination').

Approximately two-thirds of the sample were officially unrecognised as homeless. Initially they relied on family and friends for accommodation or on the private rented sector (PRS). In time, however, most of those with family and friends moved elsewhere, typically into the PRS, but a small number were then accepted by the local authority as homeless on the grounds that 'parents, relatives or friends [were] no longer willing or able to accommodate'. Thus, in time a greater proportion of those homeless due to possession are accepted as officially homeless than Table 6.1 suggested (from

Table 6.4 Housing destinations of households following possession

	Initial destination (%) (base 101)	Final destination (%) (base 101)
Family	14	7
Friends	9	1
B&B	9	3
Local authority housing	22	32
Housing association housing	3	8
Private rented housing	33	37
Bought another home	4	8
Other	6	4

Source: Ford *et al.* (1995) *Mortgage Arrears and Possessions,* London: HMSO. Own analysis

around 30 to about 40 per cent) but the route to acceptance as eligible for rehousing is not always direct, even though the underlying cause of homelessness remains constant.

The importance of the PRS for households who experience possession is clear. It is the initial destination for half of the unrecognised homeless and in time still provides for almost four out of ten of those giving possession. The PRS in respect of provision for homeless households in general is already known to be problematic (Bevan and Rhodes 1996; Chapter 13, this volume; Shelter 1996), and those entering the sector after experiencing possession share many of these problems and experiences. There are issues of access, ability to maintain rental payments, quality of accommodation and security of tenure. Following possession, ex-mortgagors may have no means of providing a deposit for the accommodation, and many are unsure of their likely eligibility for Housing Benefit. A proportion will be faced with continuing financial liabilities where their lender decides to pursue them for any shortfall on the sale of the property. One or more of these and other factors may result in considerable mobility both within and without the sector (Ford 1994). And all these issues are likely to become more pronounced with the passing of the 1996 Housing Act with its implications for the priority that can be accorded to rehousing homeless people, and the envisaged further reliance on the PRS (Shelter 1996). Problems of this nature are one of the reasons why some households, homeless through possession, return to owner occupation, either through lenders willing to provide mortgages for such households or by parents and relatives making the purchase (Ford et al. 1995).

MORTGAGE POSSESSIONS, HOMELESSNESS AND POLICY ISSUES

It might be argued that the recent increase in mortgage possessions and consequent homelessness has been a regrettable but isolated incident brought about by a particular conjunction of events that are unlikely to be repeated, not least because the mistakes made in the 1980s are now clearly recognised. The government's economic policy includes a commitment to control inflation and to prevent rapid increases in house prices and to expand labour market opportunities. Equally, lenders are concerned not to repeat the losses of the last few years and so are implementing policies whereby they expect new borrowers to have some equity in the property (by providing a deposit) and encouraging them to take out insurance against loss of income due to unemployment, accident and sickness.

While these measures are clearly important, nevertheless, housing policy remains fundamentally unchanged, focused on owner occupation and continuing to provide encouragement for people to purchase through mechanisms such as Tenants' Incentives Schemes and Voluntary Purchase Grants. The structure of provision is such that the social and private rental sectors remain limited and potentially subject to further decline, while the provision of housing *per se* is argued to be inadequate to meet projected need (Holmans 1995). All these factors make it likely that any reduction in owner occupation will be highly constrained and that marginal buyers will continue to enter.

Arguably, the risks of holding of a mortgage also remain high. Low inflation ensures that for new entrants, the initial loan-to-income ratio is not eroded, extending the period over which they are particularly exposed to risk. Average repayments as a percentage of average income have fallen from the peak in the early 1990s, but they are still approaching 20 per cent (see Table 6.2). House-price increases (in the context of new entrants holding some equity) will cushion these risks but price increases may prove to be very limited or slow to materialise. A wide range of labour market changes are also starting to impinge on mortgagors (Ford and Wilcox 1994; Ford and Wilcox 1996), many of which increase the likelihood of periods of financial disruption. In addition, the state safety net, providing assistance with mortgage interest for Income Support claimants has been severely curtailed (Ford *et al.* 1995), while the take-up of (replacement) private insurance remains low (Ford and Kempson 1997a). It is difficult therefore to escape the conclusion that although the very high levels of arrears and possessions seen in the early 1990s might not be repeated, the level of arrears is likely to remain considerable. While possession, and so homelessness, will be lower, they will also remain significant.

A number of outstanding policy issues therefore remain. Simplistically, they might be seen as dividing amongst three concerns: potential changes to the structure of provision to ensure greater housing choice and thereby limit the number of more marginal home owners; issues of assisting low-income borrowers to meet their mortgage costs and so sustain their home ownership; and ways of ensuring that those who are unable to meet their payments can secure access to alternative housing without first becoming homeless. Each of these areas is now increasingly well rehearsed, but no less important for that. Each concern has given rise to proposals – for example, for a mortgage benefit (Webb and Wilcox 1991); for mortgage rescue schemes (HACAS 1995); for flexible tenure (Terry 1996); and for the provision of new public/private safety net provisions (Wilcox and Sutherland 1997) – few if any of which have been implemented. While this situation remains, owner occupiers remain at risk of homelessness as indicated above. The challenge for housing and social policy therefore remains to develop ways of supporting those who by choice or constraint are home buyers in a social and economic system considerably less secure than it was.

Chapter 7

Soldiering on?
Theorising homelessness amongst ex-servicemen

Paul Higate

There has developed a widely held belief that as many as one-quarter of single homeless people have a background in the armed forces. This figure orginates in data collected by the Centre for Housing Policy for the Department of the Environment in 1991 (Anderson *et al.* 1993), which was subsequently the subject of secondary analysis by CRISIS (Randall and Brown 1994). Secondary analysis of the same data by the present author suggests that the efficacy of military service on predisposing ex-members of the Forces to homelessness may be somewhat overstated, partly as a consequence of the unique position the military occupies within the British psyche. Nevertheless, there is still some evidence to suggest that people with some form of military experience are overrepresented amongst people who are homeless, albeit not to the extent suggested by CRISIS. This chapter considers how some of the links between homelessness and a background in the Forces can best be conceptualised by drawing upon some of the analytic resources provided by contemporary social and cultural theory.

The chapter begins by examining the manner in which the military experience creates a profound and highly functional sense of ontological security amongst Forces personnel. It then considers how this ontological security is masculinised and how this manifests itself in the actions of servicemen. Next it considers how this masculinised ontological security creates a sense of identity which is often at odds with a civilian world increasingly pervaded by processes of individualisation and social reflexivity. Finally, it considers how this tension may feature in both the genesis and sustaining of homelessness in the case of ex-servicemen.

THE MILITARY EXPERIENCE

The military environment is one in which strong self-identity is fostered. To an outsider, shorn heads and the subsumption of individuality into a uniform mass may appear to undermine the development of a strong sense of self. This is not always so, as the military experience can create a powerful *ontological security* (Giddens 1991). For some the military experience provides a secure niche in a surrogate household. For perhaps the first time, a number of individuals establish a powerful sense of belonging. As David Morgan views it: 'there's no mention of love in the recruiting ads, but these lads have found it here; in each other's grins, in the poky, warm, muscular fug of their barrack room' (*Observer*, 24 January, 1988, cited in Morgan 1990: 26).

Similarly, the view from an Army psychiatrist illustrates that a career in the Forces is, for some, far more than a reluctant move into the world of employment: 'their [the service individual] joining the army is not simply in order to get a job, but in order to find a family which will nurture and respect them. Some of these young men find exactly that' (O'Brien 1993: 288).

Ontological security, then, is derived from a secure psychological and emotional state; as Giddens puts it, a 'confidence or trust that the natural or social worlds are as they appear to be, including the basic existential parameters of self and social identity' (Giddens 1991: 38). Confidence or trust that the world is as it appears is derived from routine as a way to buttress the self against ever threatening 'existential anxiety'. Ritual activities answer uncertainties concerning 'self and belonging' (Giddens 1984, 1991). The value of this conceptual formulation is the onus placed on continuity so that ontological security is asserted to derive from 'a sense of continuity and order in events' (Giddens 1991: 243). Ontological security in the military setting is not necessarily derived from routine in the popular sense; flowing from the well-spring of belonging may come a deep-rooted pride and profound belief that your daily task is – no matter how apparently trivial – integral to the overall functioning of the regiment, squadron or ship. Potential chaos (in the sense meant by Giddens – the omnipresent anxieties 'waiting in the wings') is banished through constant reinvestment into a particular social system that values its members through paternalistic channels.

Bourdieu, in his discussion of class, introduces some further understanding of what it means to be part of such a strong social collective. There is enormous potential power latent within – almost literally – the military 'machine'. To be part of the military parade – the synchronous movement of bodies of men – is to achieve near-flawless equilibrium: 'the practices of the same agent, and, more generally, the practices of all agents of the same [class], owe the stylistic affinity which makes each of them a metaphor of any of the others' (Bourdieu 1984: 172–3). Here aesthetic dimensions and a sense of belonging are fused. To be a serviceman is in many ways to be aware (in Giddens' existential sense), that one is – at all times and in all situations – an element of a proven whole:

> Sergeant majors bear down with huge chests and an autocratic imperative. Slim young Sergeants move with practised precision on their own or in pairs, twiddling extended pace-sticks beside the right hip like giant brass and wood dividers, though when the same Sergeants march a shaven-headed squad in double time from one place to another they appear to take on new, temporarily hysterical, personalities. Meanwhile the recruits at the bottom of the chain jerk like overwound clockwork toys; their rigidity on the command eyes right, makes them look as though they have dislocated their necks. And, even while their bodies move rapidly, they have a dazed, uncomprehending look.
>
> (Beevor 1990: 15)

The potency of this military aesthetic comes into particularly sharp focus when we consider the role of technology in modern warfare. Consider, for example, the following imagery:

> the hundreds of helicopters I'd flown in begin to draw together until they'd formed a collective meta-chopper, and in my mind it was the sexiest thing going; saver–destroyer, provider–waster, right hand–left hand, nimble fluent, canny and human; hot steel, grease, jungle-saturated canvas webbing, sweat cooling and warming up again, cassette rock and roll in one ear and door-gun fire in the other.
>
> (Herr, 1978: 77)

Servicemen – especially those working with multi-million-pound military hardware – may have direct lines to these dream-like juxtapositions.

Where in 'civvy street' can senses of belonging, of harmony and unity of the self with technology be approached? A knowledge that life can never reach these heights, that the only possible future is a civilian existence shot through with second-best adventures may jar the self. Resonance of this traumatic hiatus may be far-reaching so that past strategies are continually reinserted into current practices. Ex-servicemen may 'maintain an identification with the prior role such that the individual experiences certain aspects of the role after [he or she] has in fact exited from it' (Fuchs 1988: 6). Indeed, post-discharge hardship, such as homelessness, may invoke elements of a military persona inculcated in similarly testing circumstances.

For Giddens (1984: 36), 'practical consciousness is the cognitive and emotive anchor of the feelings on ontological security' and is analogous to the notion of 'unreflective accommodation' found in the classic work of Taylor and Cohen (1992: 47). The notion of 'habitus' found in the work of Bourdieu dovetails with these two conceptual frameworks quite neatly. For Bourdieu there is a 'practical mastery of the logic or of the imminent necessity of a game – a mastery acquired by experience of the game, and one which works outside conscious control and discourse (in the way that, for instance, techniques of the body do)' (Bourdieu 1990: 61). Thus, activities characterised by these concepts may not be discursively apparent to the agent (or in this case the serviceman) – they are 'unthinking' ways of perceiving and acting within everyday routine (Taylor and Cohen 1992; Giddens 1984, 1991). They may appear as 'habits', often with their origin in the military training context: saluting as a response to an officer; a close attention to physical appearance; distinctive ways in which to carry the military embodied self; and so on.

We can then conceptualise the serviceman's body – the military body – as the point at which man and power meld with each other. Thus, for instance, 'appearance is unusually important in the military, especially when it is accompanied by strength and agility' (Willett 1990: 15). The imperceptible characteristics of these processes channelled through the body account for their tenacity. As Bourdieu views it: 'the principles embodied in this way are placed beyond the grasp of consciousness, and hence cannot be touched by voluntary, deliberate transformation, cannot even be made explicit' (Bourdieu 1984: 93–4). For many, then, the miliary habitus remains pervasive – the self cannot fail to refer continually to the military persona. Activities encouraged to colonise the practical consciousness may take an awful lot of 'unlearning', their resonance may be far-reaching, perhaps never forgotten.

The justification for exposing the self to such concerted socialisation processes is of course often a matter of life and death. The eliciting of near-spontaneous response to orders is crystallised in the combat domain. As knowledgeable agents, servicemen are acutely aware of their finitude, the military environment is one in which reflection on dangerous duty must be tempered so as not to subvert the following of orders. Action and reaction to commands are encouraged in day-to-day activity. Similar absolute response – carried out at the level of the practical consciousness – may act as the base impetus for placing oneself in potentially catastrophic danger. The relegation of possible death to the level of the practical consciousness does not mean, however, that combat soldiers (in this case) are little more than automatons. Rather, engagement with differing levels of consciousness frees up the agent from potentially stressful (and therefore distracting) introspection. Questions (that may result in mutiny, desertion or dissent) are deterred from roaming around the discursive consciousness, sense of self is contingent on a solid understanding of what may be required. An effective serviceman – more especially combat soldiers – will almost certainly draw on an ontological security rooted in trust, hope and courage – trust in terms of the degree to which fellow soldiers' actions may be predicted; hope in the face of a body bag as one's final destination; and courage permeating the former two – rely fundamentally on the strong capabilities of the self.

Beyond initial training trust is built up during shared experiences of hardship and from trust flows hope and courage. For Giddens (1991: 38), this 'trust in others . . . is at the origin of the experience of a stable external world and a coherent sense of self-identity . . . [it is] . . . what creates a sense of ontological security . . . [and what] . . . carr[ies] the individual through transitions, crises and circumstances of high risk'. Such a theorisation helps us to grasp the pervasivity of military experience. Recognition that the realms of discursive and practical consciousness are not mutually exclusive – indeed their interface is both fluid and manipulable (Giddens 1984, 1991) – point to the importance of this area for further study in terms of the complex processes of *institutionalisation*:

conscious and unconscious mental processes lie at opposite ends of a continuum . . . in between is an area which is, as yet, little considered by sociologists . . . inasmuch as it is the domain of habit it is of great sociological importance . . . this may be where much [in this example, military] socialization put down their strongest roots . . . it is also likely to be the source of the potency of the processes of institutionalization.

(Jenkins 1992: 179)

Ontological security is fostered in an environment characterised by the direct reproduction and deployment of masculinities (Morgan 1994: 165). It is this dimension that requires further research as it may suggest the strategies through which men cope with difficulty against the back-drop of tenacious military and highly masculinised socialization processes.

TAKING IT LIKE A MAN? MILITARY SOCIALISATION AND NOTIONS OF MASCULINITY

Military service requires fit and active individuals who are able to endure protracted physical and mental hardship. Amongst combat soldiers (for example, the infantry, Royal Air Force Regiment, Royal Marines and the Special Forces) expectations and experience of tolerance to hardship are high. Tough field exercises, long runs with weighted back-packs, sleep deprivation and suffering characterise training and may underpin many hours of more 'routine' duty:

being able to take it like a man was, and continues to be, part of the military experience with its particular emphasis on a whole range of deprivations from harsh and sometimes all-embracing disciplines to cold water, hard beds and lack of sleep.

(Morgan 1990: 23).

Servicemen exposed regularly to the exigencies of the military environment may build up tolerance rooted within practical consciousness. An essential corollary of these experiences – to be found in many strands of masculine discourse (Canaan 1996; Wacquant 1995) – is the importance of 'taking it like a man'. Protestation at such extremes may be perceived as weakness in terms of the self and, if directed towards superordinates, likely to indicate a separation of the 'men from the boys'. Space in which expression of hardship is allowed to flourish may be far removed from the arena of the field exercise. Whilst complaining to one's colleague may be acceptable (and perhaps vital to bolster a flagging self), even this outlet may be somewhat constrained. Overall unit morale cannot afford to be undermined as a consequence of continued moaning. Connections between emotional display and the masculinised environment of the military are, however, apparent, and often at important moments, as Morgan (1994: 177) illustrates: 'tears are to be found at the heart of the military experience'. However, anxieties are usually given an outlet in which expression may remain non-discursive and later manifest themselves in acceptable male-orientated excesses. For example, the pressures of a tough field exercise often finds legitimised outlet in drinking binges. Hockey (1986) eloquently details the somewhat ritualised activities of 'licentious soldiery'. It is worth emphasising the thoroughgoing nature of these excesses and how they may contribute towards an ontological security which is highly masculinised.

It is in the off-duty company of work mates that excesses of drinking, fighting and bullying – crystallised in the murder of a Danish tour guide in Cyprus by three soldiers (*Daily Mail*, 29 March 1996) – reach extreme, and sometimes tragic, levels. Similarly, less anti-social, but nevertheless masculine-orientated pursuits, including womanising and body building, may constitute other leisure activities (Beevor 1990; Herr 1977; Hockey 1986). However, 'back regions' are asserted to provide not only an escape from the exercise of power, but are important for maintaining a sense of ontological security. That the military back region for the single serviceman may be infused with overtly celebrated aspects of the masculine ideal allows little space for avoiding self-identities that are not, to some extent at least, reliant on 'aggressive, threatening and deeply misogynist' (Morgan 1990: 177) perceptions of the world.

Lying at the core of the masculine ideal are issues around aggression, especially within the military setting. It is not possible to demarcate absolutely the areas in which violence is legitimate (such as combat), and areas in which it becomes unacceptable:

> if it [violence] goes too far you have to treat it seriously . . . well if they really badly damage people or property, if they start using the bottle for instance. Otherwise it's treated in a fairly tolerant fashion. Of course there's always the problem of getting mixed up with civilians, police-wise that is. Yet in a sense it's a good thing, as it keeps the spirit up, makes us more of a family.
>
> (Army officer, quoted in Hockey 1986: 149)

Within their career, many servicemen establish highly pervasive levels of masculinised ontological security. They may experience an all-embracing sense of belonging underpinned with degrees of unassailability. It almost goes without saying that a strong sense of

self-identity is rooted in high levels of worth and a favourable concept of self.

For some ex-servicemen the civilian environment may hold few
shocks. Transferable skills, living 'out' in non-military accommodation, and close connections with civilian clubs or social networks
ease the process of transition. But what happens to servicemen who
have made no provision for a civilian career or considered what
civilian life might entail? Their social networks may have been
entirely reliant on soldier colleagues, and off-base ventures may
have been infrequent. How might ontological security rooted in a
primarily masculine setting work through the self in the civilian
environment?

MILITARY AND CIVILIAN IDENTITIES

There exists a clear line between military personnel and 'others'.
Military culture contains a clear sense that civilians might contami-
nate and perhaps upset the internal equilibrium of the military
environment. For many servicemen and women, the other world –
the civilian world – may have only been experienced at a distance.
Physical and psychological isolation can often characterise the
military establishment:

> Military institutions appear to be, in a multiplicity of ways, highly
> and strongly bounded . . . the very activities associated with the
> military life, ultimately to do with the taking of life and the expo-
> sure to extreme physical danger, serve to establish an almost
> unbridgeable gulf between the world of the soldier and the world
> of the civilian . . . no civilian, it is argued repeatedly, can ever
> know what it is like.
>
> (Morgan 1994: 169)

If we consider that identity is something one comes to possess
through a number of *scripts* that constitute us as social subjects
(Gutterman 1994), then servicemen who experience high soldierly
'role centrality' (Fuchs 1988) might play to scripts which are largely
inappropriate in the civilian context. There may be a number of
scripts that require urgent reconstitution, prime amongst which will
be the scripts of masculinity – so central to the ontological security
of military life but increasingly less so in the civilian sphere. Other
military scripts may also have to be abandoned – the soldierly script
is somewhat redundant in 'civvy street' and may find expression only

within specific contexts including security work, or in the extreme, in employment as a mercenary.

Other scripts crucial to a successful civilian life also have to be acquired, foremost amongst which is the urgent necessity for people to be *reflexive*. A number of social commentators, foremost amongst whom are Giddens (1991) and Beck and Beck-Gernsheim (1996), have argued that the central feature of contemporary society is the profound shift which has occurred towards 'individualisation' processes. Their argument is that although the old sociological dictum that people make their own history (social agency) but not under conditions of their own choosing (social structures) still holds, the balance has shifted towards social agency and away from social structural determinants of social action. Beck and Beck-Gernsheim (1996: 27), for instance, argue that: 'one of the decisive features of individualization processes . . . is that they not only permit, but demand an active contribution by individuals . . . if they are not to fail individuals must be able to plan for the long term and adapt to change; they must organise and improvise, set goals, recognise obstacles, accept defeats and attempt new starts, they need initiative, tenacity, flexibility . . . '.

The hierarchical characteristics of the military structure dictate a serviceman's access to information. The 'need to know' principle ensures that knowledge (operational and of other matters) remains fragmented, and therefore, relatively secure. Ability to act is dependent on particular knowledge resources which become decreasingly circumscribed as the hierarchy is ascended. This necessarily curtails reflexivity for those situated within the lower ranks. Indeed, high dependence levels are encouraged, as the institution remains the prime site from which crucial information flows. Accommodation, food, on- and off-duty dress codes, official tasks and broadly consensual world views provide guiding channels along which reflexivity is encouraged to run.

Issues of identity may therefore become a problematic issue for some ex-servicemen and anomie may characterise their striving for secure and familiar scripts. Within the military setting, internal contradiction in terms of the discursive production of subjects (the soldierly role) is minimised. For example, incompetence and femininity are asserted to go hand-in-hand (Hockey 1986), thereby exemplifying the potency of binary oppositions in the constitution of identity. However, if we focus on the discursive aspects of identity in the civilian context, it becomes clear that there are conflicts among discursive systems and contradictions and ambiguities within any one of them.

Themes of ontological security, masculinised socialisation and institutionalisation characterise the prime tenets of this analytic framework and offer some insights into links between service in the Armed Forces and homelessness. However, this remains only part of the picture. Taken together, these concepts should point towards a generative mechanism (military/masculine socialisation) that predisposes individuals to a particular form of social exclusion (homelessness). That a significant majority of ex-servicemen do not experience homelessness does not mean that they remain untouched by this intensive process, but nevertheless leads us to consider other factors, including non-military experience. In considering this framework, we should also consider the temporal dimension. In this way notions of institutionalisation and its far-reaching resonance can be conceptualised over the entire life-course.

PRE-MILITARY EXPERIENCE

There is a tendency to see military experience as the most significant element of any biography. The media, and in particular the tabloids, remain preoccupied with military experience when reporting crimes from rape to burglary. In a number of ways this returns us to the largely latent (though potent) position the military occupies within British society. In theorising homelessness, then, it may be better to consider the military experience as one of a number jostling for influence throughout a particular life-cycle. Jolly's (1996) work focused on the transition from the military to the civilian environment. She found that many were able to move quickly from the experience with future activities drawing on current energies, and the military past destined for little more than nostalgic indulgence.

Fieldwork currently being carried out by the author points to the importance of experiences prior to enlistment. Three ex-servicemen describe elements of their life shortly before joining up:

> I could do more or less what I wanted and when you're 14 or 15 you think it's great . . . it ended up [mum] wasn't paying rent . . . so we got evicted. It didn't bother me, you know – out on't streets – there used to be a caravan . . . it was a case of I used to climb over the fence and go there at night, get the blankets out and sleep there.
>
> (Dave, 43, three years' Army service)

I was bought up in Moss Side, know what I mean? We were
bought up in the slums and all that, which was a bit of training for
us as well . . . you get your dinner cooked for you every Sunday
an' all that then you've gotta go out there all the time, so we
weren't watching television like the kids nowadays, and watching
computers an' all that, for one of them to go outside and survive,
they haven't got the training to do it.

(Doug, early 30s, a 'few months in Army')

Left home when I was 14 and . . . living in a tent in the Peak District at Woodhead . . . still going to school every morning . . . 'I
was sleeping in a maggot farm at night'.

(Marko, 45, eight years' service in the Army)

Adventure, self-reliance and parental absence thread these brief
narrative excerpts together. Joining the Army developed from these
orientations and experiences of the world, with the military envisaged as the ideal environment in which the anxieties could be both
appeased through membership of the military 'family' (ontological
security), fused with excitement and responsibility. The relevance of
pre-military experience in homeless Vietnam veterans has also been
shown to be significant. Evidence suggests that substance abuse and
familial mental health problems prior to conscription may have been
significant in disposing these people to later homelessness (Rosenheck and Fontana 1994; Wenzel *et al.* 1993).

TAKING IT LIKE A 'CIVVY'

Feelings that a great pressure has been lifted may characterise the
experience of many servicemen on discharge. The move to the civilian
world may be one of the most enlightening processes to befall the individual. For some it is an escape from a claustrophobic environment
that robs individuality and thwarts independence. Perhaps a job has
been lined up and the aftermath of the military experience is akin to a
'honeymoon period'. No more uniform, no more feeling like an
extremely small cog in a grindingly powerful machine. Decisions pro-
liferate concerning payment of utility bills, shopping for food, cooking, ignoring the possibility that one's car may have been targeted by
the IRA, space to move, space to think, freedom!

Or perhaps things are not quite as one expected, if one expected
anything at all. How does one pay a bill? Where is the water meter?

Do I need a TV licence? How much is it? Electricity, gas, the DSS, prescription charges, clothing for work, how am I expected to dress . . . ? Out-of-town shopping at a distant supermarket, paying to join a gym? Renting a place? Friends?

Ontological security fostered in the military environment has been shown – for some at least – to be of profound importance; its links with institutionalisation (which in the majority of cases may not lead to social exclusion) should be evident. However, also highlighted are the weaker links between the military experience and homelessness. Hitherto, notions of institutionalisation have been loosely applied and under-theorised. The concept is almost always used negatively and devoid of its obvious gender and temporal dimensions. In theorising homelessness amongst ex-servicemen generally, we can look briefly at Jock, who served nine years in the Army.

Though Jock's military career could hardly be described as exemplary (with spells in the glasshouse for brawling), he left the Army married and with two young children. The death of his wife and sister sparked a series of events culminating in homelessness. His story reads much like many other homeless individuals: tragedy, inability to cope, problematic relationship to alcohol, and so forth. However, it is only now (after nine years in and out of prison, rough sleeping and excessive drinking) that Jock recognises the influence the Army had on his civilian life. A period of five years elapsed before homelessness appeared – up until then, the Army had apparently been put firmly behind him. However, a deep-rooted pride fostered in the military was fresh in Jock's mind:

> You used to have talks with the Padre [Army chaplain], you were always that bit wary that someone was gonna find out – because in the Army – everybody has their eyes on each other and if you thought a guy had a weakness, you wanted to stay well away from that guy . . . it leads to a snowball effect . . . 'this fucker's no right in the head' . . . it got that way . . . before long they'd be out of the Army.

When problems struck, his response (inertia at best, solace sought through the bottle at worse) served to sustain homelessness: 'No, no, you try not to get help, you try desperately to resolve your own problems . . . even now a' still . . . to a certain extent . . . you still feel you've gotta be in control – if you're not in control it's as if you've failed.'

A recently discharged soldier, with service in Northern Ireland and the Gulf, writes the following:

I hate asking for help, but on this occasion [becoming homeless] I really needed it . . . what about all those squaddies who are too proud to ask for help? This is not 1 or 2 – it's bred into you when you are in the Army . . . to get on with it, just do it, stop whinge-ing etc . . . you must understand that a squaddie will see asking for help as a weakness.

(Letter to author, February 1996)

Of course pride is not unique to the homeless ex-serviceman; indeed, it is a powerful theme expressed by many of those like the homeless with a pariah-like status. However, when it is combined with tolerance to hardship, there exists a readily accessible cluster of discourses (or scripts) through which homelessness may be 'dealt with'. First the experience of being cold and wet, and sleep-ing on a hard surface may not be so foreign. Second and crucially, it may be conceptualised at the level of practical consciousness as a 'quasi-challenge'. Ways in which masculinised ontological security buttressed the self within the military context may resurface and become manifest in the tough embodied ability of the self to overcome a testing situation. For example, commenting on a week's spell of homelessness, an ex-soldier with three years' service said:

To tell you the truth it didn't bother me . . . . I just looked at it like doing a fieldcraft exercise . . . something like that . . . yeah . . . . I just like slept in bushes . . . it was summertime, it was all right, it wasn't cold, I just slept in bushes, sheds, you know . . . a new experience . . . wouldn't like to do it again.

Marko also recalls sleeping rough: 'it would have been harder for me, if I wasn't in the Forces, you know what I mean, it would have been harder for me, because I'm used to the cold and all that, the cold doesn't bother me now.'
And Dave:

In a way it helped [being in the Army] because you used to do the old training exercises, where you went out so, I was lucky in the respect that I got a sleeping bag, so it wasn't too bad, so yeah . . . it sort of, how can I put it, not toughens you but it prepares you for anything like that, you know if you have to sleep out.

On the face of it, these soldiers made a 'choice' to sleep rough. Choice, however, requires explication. There was no active decision to seek help, because the notion of need remained elusive to the self.

The legacy of the military experience intervened so as not to problematise sleeping rough. Indeed, the colonisation of the practical consciousness with routine learned in the military (or perhaps before, but certainly reinforced in this environment) may further infuse self-worth and bolster a threatened self-esteem.

CONCLUDING COMMENT

The temptation to conflate military service and homelessness is great. This tendency flows from the largely mythologised perceptions surrounding the military institution and its apparent production of 'unthinking automatons'. In theorising homelessness amongst ex-servicemen, we have shown the extent to which some agents are drawn into a particular masculinised total institution. It is this minor-ity – characterised perhaps by their early trajectory of relative disad-vantage and instability – that may perceive the military as a 'way out' of hardship, and a way in to a 'family'.

Themes of ontological security and the temporal/gender dynamics of institutionalisation have been highlighted. It is likely that their effects have greatest significance for homeless ex-servicemen, and the chapter should be considered with these individuals in mind. Pre-military experience has been briefly considered, together with the crucial notion of pride and tolerance to hardship. Provision seeking may be characterised by a contradictory mix of genuine need infused with a reluctance to admit what is constituted by the self as 'weak-ness'. Though provisional fieldwork suggests that pathways into homelessness for ex-servicemen tend not to differ substantially from those of their non-service homeless cohort, behaviour when socially excluded may do. Furthermore, it is premised (notably for those with experience in higher-status military occupations such as the Special Forces), a civilian existence can only ever be second best. In this way it is helpful to consider degrees of 'integration' or anomie on dis-charge from the military, with homelessness appearing at the starkest and most extreme pole.

Chapter 8

The housing needs of ex-prisoners[1]

Jane Carlisle

The housing situation of ex-prisoners is an important issue that affects both those people who are released from prison and society as a whole. Recent research on accommodation for ex-prisoners is scarce, but it has been demonstrated (Banks and Fairhead 1976) that 66 per cent of homeless ex-prisoners re-offend within twelve months of release, compared with 22 per cent of those who retain or acquire accommodation.

The aims of the study reported in this chapter were to examine: first, ex-prisoners' experiences of pre-release information on accommodation; second, the difficulties that ex-prisoners face in finding and keeping temporary and permanent accommodation; and third, providers' perceptions of the housing needs of ex-prisoners and the provision made for them. The chapter begins with a review of the methodology used for the research and moves on to discuss the numbers of ex-prisoners who are in housing need. The chapter then examines the provision of services for ex-prisoners with regard to finding and keeping accommodation, and concludes with a discussion of how the current range of services could be improved.

THE RESEARCH

The research was composed of three elements. First, semi-structured interviews were conducted with prisoners who were about to be released. The prisoners were asked whether they had received any housing information while they were in prison, and if they would be willing to participate in the follow-up phase of the research. One hundred and thirty-four interviews were carried out with male prisoners and 41 with female prisoners, giving a total of 175 interviews in total. Prisoners were interviewed in eight prisons spread across the country. Second, semi-structured interviews were conducted with probation officers and providers of accommodation for ex-prisoners, from both the statutory and voluntary sectors. Third, semi-structured interviews were conducted with a follow-up sample taken from the prisoners who had been interviewed in the first phase. The semi-structured interviews were conducted between four and eight months after the prisoners' discharge from prison. The ex-prisoners were asked about their experiences in finding and keeping suitable accommodation and the usefulness of any information they had received about finding accommodation while still in prison. At this stage, thirty-seven male prisoners and twelve female prisoners were interviewed, giving forty-nine interviews in total. In twelve cases interviews were obtained with the relatives of ex-prisoners, when the ex-prisoners themselves could not be contacted.

HOW MANY EX-PRISONERS ARE IN HOUSING NEED?

Around 100,000 prisoners are released from prisons every year in England and Wales (Home Office 1995). However, no statutory statistics are kept on the numbers of prisoners who are released without suitable housing to go to, and no other data are currently available.[2] It is therefore difficult to estimate how many released prisoners have no satisfactory accommodation. There has been little recent work carried out on the housing needs of ex-prisoners apart from the research undertaken by Paylor (1992) in Lancaster. Paylor found that just over half of the sixty-eight ex-prisoners he interviewed approximately two weeks after their release (51.4 per cent) had experienced a negative change in their accommodation compared with their housing before they were imprisoned. Paylor found that 40 per cent of prisoners were released to no fixed abode, a figure comparable with that in the present study, which found that seventy-five ex-prisoners (43 per cent) had no accommodation on discharge. These figures may not be representative, but if they were typical, a crude 'guesstimate' can be produced which suggests that in excess of some 40,000 prisoners could, currently, be released each year without having any pre-arranged accommodation to go to.[3]

CURRENT PRACTICE

Services provided on discharge

A standard discharge grant or a higher discharge grant was given to prisoners at the time of their release. At the time the research was conducted, the standard grant was £36.15 for people aged 16 to 24 and £45.70 for people aged 25 and over (Hagell *et al.* 1995). In theory, the grant provided a substitute for one week of Income Support. All discharged prisoners were entitled to this grant (unless they were actually in employment at the time of release – for example, on a pre-release work scheme). Prisoners who were released to no fixed abode qualified for the higher discharge grant, which nominally included a week's Housing Benefit and a standard discharge grant, totalling £91.65.

The extra money given to prisoners released to no fixed abode was seen by many prisoners who had access to accommodation as an incentive to practise deception about their housing situation on release. Prisoners could receive more than double the amount of the standard discharge grant simply by saying they had nowhere to live. The attraction of the higher-rate discharge grant might be interpreted as possibly distorting the results of research into housing need among ex-prisoners. However, during the course of the research, the difficulty in securing a higher discharge grant was increasing. The introduction of devolved prison budgets in April 1994 gave prison governors responsibility for all expenditure within their prison. According to a number of the prison staff who were interviewed, some governors quickly became aware that the higher discharge grant was an area in which it would be possible to make savings without suffering any loss regarding the normal regime or activities within the prison. It appeared that in many prisons a default system of allowing only the standard discharge grant had become a key area for saving money. The onus was placed on the prisoner to prove, commonly by corroboration from their home probation officer, that they had no accommodation to go to in order to qualify for the higher discharge grant.[4] Statistics on discharge grants were not available at the time the research was conducted.

Another criterion used by prison staff in deciding whether or not a prisoner would be homeless on release was based on where they had resided for pre-release home leave. Home leave is granted to prisoners who are serving a sentence of over six months; this temporary release from prison on parole is part of the rehabilitation programme designed to enable them to re-enter mainstream society successfully. Often, prison staff assumed that any prisoner who had provided a private address (rather than a hostel address) at which they had spent a pre-release home leave could reside there on discharge. However, this was frequently demonstrated to have been an erroneous assumption when interviews were conducted with prisoners several months after release. Many ex-prisoners stated that parents, relatives or friends who were willing to have them stay for a few days were unwilling to provide them with permanent accommodation.

Services provided in the community for ex-prisoners

Since data on the extent to which ex-prisoners are able to access suitable accommodation on discharge are not collected on any scale, it is not possible to estimate what the prevalence of homelessness among ex-offenders might be. The present study and Paylor (1992) found high levels of housing need among prisoners at the point of discharge and strong evidence that this situation persisted for some ex-prisoners for months. There are also some data that indicate that at least some ex-prisoners join the single homeless population. Anderson *et al.* (1993: 32) found that 4 per cent of single homeless men reported that their last accommodation had been prison.

Although most ex-prisoners who were interviewed in the follow-up phase had tried to acquire homes, many had been unsuccessful. People released from prison rarely had enough money on which to survive until they could receive benefit, and were unable to raise a deposit with which to secure a private tenancy. Few ex-prisoners were able to arrange accommodation purely by their own efforts.

Housing need is, of course, relative. The probation officers who were interviewed in the second phase of the study were almost unanimous in their view that they could find a bed for the night for every discharged prisoner. Thus, it could be argued that there is no unmet need in relation to accommodation for ex-prisoners, if the quality of the accommodation is disregarded. However, the accommodation that could be arranged by Probation was often in B&B or shared hostel accommodation and met only the most basic and short-term forms of housing need. Very few prisoners were willing to be discharged to such accommodation, although some had no option when it was a condition of their parole licence.

Two forms of hostel accommodation are provided for ex-offenders. A number of hostels are operated directly by the Home Office and are designed to accommodate people on probation or a parole licence, as well as individuals on bail. They function according to strict rules, including a curfew, and are seen as providing an alternative to custody as well as having a role in accommodating ex-prisoners. Some voluntary organisations and housing associations also run hostels for offenders with funding from the Home Office. These schemes tend to be targeted at ex-prisoners who are vulnerable, such as people with a mental health problem, and provide care and support services as well as elements of resettlement (for a general discussion of hostels for homeless people, see Neale, this volume).

Probation officers took the view that hostels, through their links with other agencies and their resettlement services, could function as a 'stepping stone' that would allow ex-prisoners to secure permanent accommodation. Ex-prisoners, however, had a very different view of hostels, some criticising conditions within such accommodation as 'worse than prison'. Two factors were paramount in prisoners' dislike of hostels. The first was that most, if not all, of the other residents in the hostel were ex-offenders; indeed, very often residents were offending while in the hostel, which created a poor, and sometimes threatening, atmosphere. From what the prisoners said, the dominant visual feature of many hostels was squalor. They were described as not only unacceptably dirty, with reference to the communal areas such as the lavatories, bathrooms and kitchens, but nauseating because of the evidence of drug abuse, such as used hypodermic needles and vomit. People who are under the influence of drugs can be extremely difficult and unpleasant, and sometimes dangerous to deal with. Some prisoners who participated in the study were determined to make an effort to remain drug-free after their release, and explained the virtual impossibility of achieving this when they had nothing to do, were living in the miserable circumstances of a hostel and were offered drugs.

Not all hostels suffered from the problems described above. Some were kept in good order, with little dispute between residents, who nevertheless found conditions in the hostel irksome because of what they perceived as many petty rules. These rules typically included bans on alcohol and drugs, no guests being allowed on the premises and a curfew. For all or some of the above reasons, a large number of ex-prisoners preferred to be 'homeless' rather than accept a place in a hostel.

Alternatives to hostel accommodation were often difficult to find. Ex-prisoners were unlikely to have access to local authority accommodation because they were not considered to be 'vulnerable'. Few ex-prisoners can access the private rented sector, as provision of a bond or rent in advance was beyond the means of the vast majority (Rugg, this volume). Several prisoners who were interviewed had written either to their local authority housing department or to a local housing association, or both, in the expectation of going on a waiting list so that they might be housed on, or soon after, their discharge from prison. However, the response from local authorities and housing associations had been the same in every case: while in prison people were not considered to be in housing need, and therefore could not be placed on a housing waiting list before they had been discharged from custody. Former prisoners who continued to apply for social housing after their release were usually unsuccessful.

A number of local authorities had provided housing for ex-prisoners very soon after their discharge from prison. This was invariably in spare accommodation, in what are sometimes described as 'low demand areas'. This housing was offered to those ex-prisoners who were classed as single and not vulnerable, apparently because the properties would otherwise have remained unoccupied. The accommodation was often surrounded by many houses that were boarded up, where paths and roads were littered with broken glass and other rubbish and other inhabited properties appeared to be in a poor condition. The ex-prisoners in the study who had accepted social housing in a low demand area faced huge problems. Initially, they had difficulty in furnishing their homes on inadequate grants or loans from the Social Fund.[5] Apart from the inadequately furnished interior of the accommodation, and the typical squalor of the near environment, such low demand areas were, the ex-prisoners said, frightening places in which to live because of 'joyriders', people smashing windows and other types of vandalism.

One local authority in the study had an implicit policy of including ex-prisoners under the heading of 'vulnerable' people. They had not made the policy explicit because of the antagonism it might generate from local residents in an area that already suffered from a high level of drug dealing and vandalism. Nevertheless, the staff who were interviewed expressed a view that people leaving prison needed support, and especially good-quality housing, in order to provide them with the opportunity of rebuilding a life without resorting to re-offending.

CONCLUDING COMMENTS

The first step to producing an integrated and effective housing policy in relation to ex-prisoners would be to introduce a single amount standard discharge grant. The grant should be available to all prisoners on discharge regardless of their age or housing situation, and should be sufficient to provide for ex-prisoners until they can claim benefit.

An effective policy would start with practical advice being a part of the prisoners' reception programme on entering prison to help them to retain existing accommodation. For those prisoners who have lost accommodation, an integrated system of service delivery requiring inter-agency collaboration between prison staff, voluntary sector providers of accommodation, local authority housing departments and housing associations should be established. This group of agencies might best be co-ordinated by a housing specialist from the Probation Service in the prisoner's home area.

A desolate picture of hostels has been painted, as seen through the eyes of some prisoners who were interviewed. An outcome of the unpopularity of hostels is that, as people are so reluctant to reside in them, many hostels house fewer residents than their capacity. Many hostels are partly or wholly funded by the Home Office, which applies strict criteria regarding the occupancy rate of hostels. The minimum allowable occupancy rate over a year for hostels to maintain their grant is 75 per cent. Many hostels have found it difficult to achieve this level of occupancy, and in some hostels staff are deployed to chase referrals.

Traditional hostel accommodation is no longer acceptable as satisfactory housing. However, the good practice on which a review of unsatisfactory hostel provision might draw is already in evidence within the housing association sector. Some voluntary organisations engaged in providing hostel accommodation have taken an innovative approach. These organisations have decreased the number of beds in their hostels, and have acquired properties, usually two-bedroom terrace houses, within a short distance of hostel buildings. The hostel then becomes known as 'core' accommodation, and the small houses as 'cluster' accommodation. A resident goes first to the main hostel, for assessment, and if it is appropriate, they may quickly be allocated a place in one of the cluster houses, sharing with one other person and with visits, usually once or twice a week, from staff. Those ex-prisoners who are seen as needing more support, often in what may be thought of as ordinary skills such as maintaining hygiene, shopping, budgeting and cooking, will stay for a longer period in the main hostel until they demonstrate an ability to cope with what amounts to independent living.

Many ex-prisoners have problems in executing such everyday tasks, simply because they have never been taught how to manage a household or even experienced a typical home environment. These problems are often exacerbated by relative poverty, loneliness and anxiety about coping on their own. This group may benefit from daily support, which could be tailored to their needs, so that support could be increased or diminished as appropriate. This form of 'floating' support may be the optimum means of helping vulnerable ex-prisoners towards independent living. When a resident is able to cope without support, instead of having to move to different accommodation, perhaps to an unfamiliar area, they can remain in their original accommodation and build on their existing relationships.

Local authority and housing association accommodation was seen by many of the ex-prisoners who were interviewed as their preferred tenure. Some prisoners are eager to plan for their future, and see adequate housing as fundamental. They would be encouraged by a more positive response from local authorities and housing associations, instead of a blanket refusal to place them on a waiting list. The great majority wish to return to what was their home area, and this would be facilitated by housing departments and the Probation Service working towards finding a constructive housing solution for ex-prisoners. It is important for parents released from prison without housing to have satisfactory accommodation as quickly as possible so that they may be reunited with their children.

NOTES

1 Material for this chapter is drawn from a study which was funded by the Joseph Rowntree Foundation and carried out by the Centre for Housing Policy at the University of York. The study began in January 1994 and was completed in September 1995. Fuller details of the study can be found in Carlisle (1996).
2 NACRO expect to produce statistics on the housing situation of released prisoners in the future.
3 Forty-three per cent may be considered to be a likely maximum proportion of prisoners released without accommodation rather than a likely average figure, because of several confounding variables. The uncertainty of prisoners, in some cases, about their welcome from family and friends on their release was an incalculable factor: a large proportion of prisoners were simply unsure whether or not they would be allowed to

resume residence in their former home. Parents, for example, might no longer wish to be responsible for their adolescent or adult offspring; a partner might have ended their relationship and retained possession or disposed of their joint home. Another factor which may have confounded the attempt to determine the number of prisoners released with no accommodation to go to was the discharge grant, as discussed.

4 Governors can reclaim moneys paid to prisoners as grants, so it is not truly money 'saved'.

5 The largest amount offered to any ex-prisoner in the study was £260.

Chapter 9

The health of single homeless people[1]

Wendy Bines

Although it is generally recognised that homelessness and poor health are related, it is difficult to demonstrate this empirically. This chapter presents evidence about the physical and mental health of single homeless people and their access to primary health care – a topic taken up in more detail in Pleace and Quilgars (this volume). The findings are based on secondary analysis of two data sources of self-reported health. The first source of data came from a national large-scale survey of single homeless people carried out in 1991. The aim of this survey was to provide information on the characteristics of single homeless people (Kemp, this volume), their reasons for becoming homeless and their accommodation needs and preferences. In total the survey involved structured interviews with three different samples of single homeless people – 1,346 people living in hostels and bed and breakfast accommodation (B&Bs) and 507 people who were sleeping rough using day centres and soup runs.[2] The second source of data came from the first wave of the British Household Panel Survey (BHPS). This is an annual survey of a nationally representative sample of at least 5,000 households and 10,000 individuals. The first wave of this study was also carried out in 1991.

Although the survey of single homeless people and the BHPS were designed and carried out independently, respondents in both surveys were asked about the same health problems. The comparison with the general population in relation to these health problems illustrates the considerably worse health of single homeless people. The findings in this chapter are important for three main reasons. First, they are based on a large national survey of single homeless people, whereas previous studies have tended to focus on single homeless people in specific geographical areas. Many studies have also focused on single homeless people using particular hostels or health services.

Second, the survey was the largest to be carried out since the late 1970s. It is, therefore, an important contemporary source of information about single homeless people and their health. Third, the availability of data from the first wave of the BHPS provided an opportunity to directly compare the self-reported health of a representative sample of single homeless people with a representative sample of the general population. This is the first time that it has been possible specifically to compare the health of single homeless people in England with that of the general population.[3]

THE PHYSICAL HEALTH OF SINGLE HOMELESS PEOPLE

Compared with the general population, single homeless people were more likely to have health problems. They were also more likely to have *more* than one health problem (Table 9.1). More than a third of people in hostels and B&Bs, and well over half the people sleeping rough, reported more than one health problem compared with a quarter of the general population. Table 9.1 also illustrates clearly that people sleeping rough experience the worst health of all.

The proportion of single homeless people and the general population who reported specific health problems are shown in Table 9.2. This shows that almost all the health problems were reported by a higher proportion of people in hostels and B&Bs than the general population, and all but one of the health problems were reported by more people sleeping rough than other single homeless people and the general population.

Table 9.1 Percentage of people reporting health problems, all ages

	Hostels & B&Bs (%)	People sleeping rough		General population (%)
		Day centres (%)	Soup runs (%)	
No health problems	38	22	24	45
One health problem	24	22	17	31
More than one health problem	38	57	59	24
(Base)	(1,280)	(351)	(156)	(10,264)

Sources: Single Homeless People Survey data (1991) and British Household Panel Survey data (1991). Own analysis

Table 9.2 Percentage of people reporting specific health problems, all ages[1]

| Health problem | Hostels and B&Bs (%) | Sleeping rough | | |
		Day centres (%)	Soup runs (%)	General population (%)
Musculoskeletal problems[2]	24	36	42	23
Difficulty in seeing	10	19	17	7
Difficulty in hearing	10	12	10	7
Wounds, skin ulcers/ complaints	10	16	19	10
Chronic chest or breathing problems	18	23	28	10
Heart problems	5	5	5	12
Digestive problems	9	12	12	6
Depression, anxiety or nerves	28	36	40	5
Fits or loss of consciousness[3]	5	13	13	1
Frequent headaches	16	17	19	8
(Base)	(1,280)	(351)	(155)	(10,264)

Sources: Single Homeless People Survey data (1991) and BHPS data (1991). Own analysis

Notes:
[1]   Definitions are those used in the survey of single homeless people
[2]   Two of the health problems ('difficulty in walking' and 'painful muscles or joints') used in the survey of single homeless people were combined in order to provide a comparison with one of the health problems ('problems or disability connected with arms, legs etc') used in the BHPS. The term 'musculoskeletal problems' is used to incorporate the definitions used in both surveys
[3]   The figures for this health problem should be treated with caution because of the different definitions used; the survey of single homeless people used 'fits or loss of consciousness' while the BHPS used the definition 'epilepsy'

Although Tables 9.1 and 9.2 provide useful information on the *absolute* percentages of people reporting health problems, their usefulness is limited as they are likely to be influenced by the differences in the age and gender structure of the survey samples. For example, whereas the general population consists of almost equal numbers of men and women, there are far fewer women among single homeless people than men. Because age and gender are two important factors known to be associated with variations in health, it was important that the data were standardised by these two factors in order that a more accurate comparison could be made between the health of single homeless people and the general population. Indirect standardisation was used to produce a standardised morbidity rate (SMR) for each of the health problems.[4] Table 9.3 shows the SMRs for each of the nine health problems summarised in Table 9.4.

In the categories shown, the prevalence of health problems in the general population is represented by the number 100. Where the figure is higher than 100, this means that the rate at which a health problem occurs was greater than the level found in the general population (150 means single homeless people are 1.5 times more likely than the general population to have a specific health problem, and so forth). Most of the health problems were two or three times higher among

Table 9.3 Standardised morbidity rates[1] (SMRs) of reported health problems[2]

	Hostels and B&Bs SMR	Sleeping rough	
		Day centres SMR	Soup runs SMR
Health problem			
Musculoskeletal problems[3]	153	185	221
Difficulty in seeing	166	313	308
Difficulty in hearing	148	163	166
Wounds, skin ulcers or other skin complaints	105	189	298
Chronic chest or breathing problems	183	259	365
Heart problems	54	64	66
Digestive problems	183	244	265
Depression, anxiety or nerves	785	1,072	1,152
Fits or loss of consciousness[4]	651	2,109	1,892
Frequent headaches	264	338	365

Sources: Single Homeless People Survey data (1991) and BHPS data (1991). Own analysis

Notes:
[1] Standardised by age and gender. The figures should be interpreted as follows: a value of 100 indicates no difference between the rate of health problems among single homeless people and the general population; a value above 100 indicates that the health of single homeless people is worse than that of the general population; and a value below 100 indicates that their health is better. For example, a value of 500 would mean that the health of homeless people is five times worse than the general population
[2] Definitions are those used in the CHP (1991) Single Homeless People Survey
[3,4] See corresponding notes to Table 9.2

Table 9.4 The health of single homeless people compared to that of the general population

Compared to the general population

- *chronic chest condition or breathing problems* were:
    - twice as high among people in hostels and B&Bs
    - three times as high as among people sleeping rough
- *heart problems* were consistently lower among homeless people
- *wounds, skin ulcers or other skin complaints* were:
    - similar among people in hostels and B&Bs
    - twice as high among people using day centres
    - three times as high among people using soup runs
- *musculoskeletal problems* were:
    - twice as high among people sleeping rough
- *difficulty in seeing* was:
    - three times as high among people sleeping rough
- *fits or loss of consciousness* were much higher among homeless people
- *digestive problems* were:
    - twice as high among people in hostels and B&Bs
    - at least twice as high as among people sleeping rough
- *frequent headaches* were:
    - at least twice as high among people in hostels and B&Bs
    - at least three times as high among people sleeping rough
- *mental health problems* were:
    - eight times as high among people in hostels and B&Bs
    - eleven times as high among people sleeping rough.

single homeless people compared with the general population. The only health problem that had a similar incidence to the general population was 'wounds, skin ulcers and other skin complaints', but this only applied to people in hostels and B&Bs – those sleeping rough were two or three times more likely than the general population to have this health problem.

The prevalence of all the health problems was higher among people sleeping rough than among those in hostels and B&Bs and the general population, thus emphasising their poorer health. Although many people interviewed in hostels and B&Bs had slept rough in the previous twelve months, this was for shorter periods than people interviewed at day centres or soup runs (Anderson *et al.* 1993). 'Chronic chest or breathing problems' were particularly high among people sleeping rough – they were two or three times more likely to suffer from this compared with the general population. In addition, people at soup runs were twice as likely, and those at day centres were almost twice as likely, to suffer from musculoskeletal problems compared with the general population.

These findings support the point made by Anderson *et al.* (1993) that the health problems more commonly found among those sleeping rough, such as chest problems, skin complaints and musculoskeletal problems, are the type of problems that could be made worse or more difficult to clear up *because* the sufferer was sleeping rough. Lack of sleep was also something that people sleeping rough felt affected their health.

Digestive problems were also prevalent among single homeless people: those in hostels were almost twice as likely to suffer from them and those sleeping rough were two and a half times more likely to report this problem than the general population. Although cheap meals are available in many hostels and day centres, and despite the free food available from soup runs, this does not mean that single homeless people are eating the well-balanced, nutritious diet that is essential for good health. A healthy diet may be difficult for homeless people to maintain for a number of reasons – including lack of money and an irregular lifestyle, making it impossible to plan the next meal. Digestive problems can be related to other health problems, and there are many factors including heavy drinking, drug dependencies and depression that can work against the maintenance of a healthy diet. Some homeless people also said they needed to eat special diets, and this was a problem for them because some hostels were unable to cater for their special needs.

The prevalence of 'difficulty in seeing' and 'difficulty in hearing' was higher among single homeless people; difficulty in seeing was particularly high among those sleeping rough, who were three times more likely to report it than the general population. This is an important finding because these are the sort of health problems that could be detected by a health check. Also it is not known whether homeless people have difficulties in using opticians or whether this is a particular problem that needs to be addressed.

The proportion of single homeless people who reported suffering from fits or loss of consciousness was very high, especially in comparison to the proportion of the general population who reported suffering from epilepsy (Table 9.2). The explanation for this higher prevalence is not clear since homelessness in itself is unlikely to be the cause. However, the majority of single homeless people who reported fits or loss of consciousness also had either alcohol-related problems, mental health problems or, to a lesser extent, drug dependencies (or a combination of all three). One in ten of those sleeping rough who reported fits said this caused them difficulty in finding or keeping accommodation.

The only health problem that was consistently lower among single homeless people was 'heart problems'.[5] The reason for this is not clear. However, a 'heart problem' is not generally a condition one would know one had without the benefit of medical advice, unlike, for example, 'frequent headaches'. Some single homeless people may have reported health problems related to heart conditions such as 'difficulty in walking' or 'breathing problems' but may not have known the underlying cause. There is also the issue of access to health services, and, given the difficulties that some homeless people are known to have in gaining access to primary health care, it may be that some homeless people have heart problems that have not been diagnosed. In addition, the low rate of heart problems among single homeless people may be due to the younger age of the sample. Heart disease predominately occurs in people over the age of fifty. The fact that homelessness carries a high risk of dying before this age (Keyes and Kennedy 1992), may explain the attenuation of heart disease among people who are homeless.

THE MENTAL HEALTH OF SINGLE HOMELESS PEOPLE

In recent years there has been increasing concern about the mental health of single homeless people, particularly those sleeping rough. For example, in 1990 the London Homeless Mentally Ill Initiative was set up, with funding from the Department of Health and the Mental Health Foundation, to provide services to homeless mentally ill people. There has also been considerable research into the mental health of single homeless people, much of which has highlighted the prevalence of mental illness among them (Timms and Fry 1989; Marshall 1989). One of the major problems of research in this area, however, is the difficulty of comparing the mental health of homeless people with that of the general population. The findings from this study are, therefore, particularly important as the same definition of self-reported mental illness, 'depression, anxiety and nerves', was used in both surveys, thus allowing a comparison to be made.

Mental health problems were much higher among single homeless people; this was reported by 28 per cent of people in hostels and B&Bs, 36 per cent of day-centre users and 40 per cent of soup-run users, compared to 5 per cent of the general population (Table 9.5). Taking into account the effect of age and gender, eight times as many people in hostels and B&Bs, and eleven times as many people sleeping rough reported mental health problems compared to the general population (Table 9.5). In addition, one in eight people in hostels and B&Bs, one in five at day centres and one in six people at soup runs had stayed in a psychiatric hospital at some time in the past (Anderson *et al.* 1993).[6]

In the general population the incidence of mental health problems increased with age; in other words, the older people are the more likely they are to have mental health problems. Among single homeless people, however, those aged between 25 and 59 years were the most likely to report mental health problems. But, relative to the general population, younger people, especially those who were sleeping rough, appear to be the most adversely affected by mental health problems. This finding emphasises the vulnerability of young homeless people. It is also an important finding because, whereas it is thought that depression is more common in the elderly than in any other age group (DoH 1993), this study shows that among single homeless people depression is actually more common among people of middle age and is relatively higher among young homeless people compared with the general population.

People sleeping rough were the most likely to have mental health

Table 9.5 Percentage of people reporting mental health problems

	Hostels & B&Bs (%)	Day centres (%)	Soup runs (%)	General population (%)
Gender				
Women	33	44	55	7
Men	26	36	37	3
Age group				
16–24	22	31	45	3
25–59	34	37	41	5
60 and over	19	29	18	7
All	28	36	40	5
(Base)	(1,280)	(351)	(156)	(10,264)

Sources: CHP Single Homeless People Survey data (1991) and BHPS data. Own analysis

problems and to have ever stayed in a psychiatric hospital. Even those in hostels and B&Bs who had slept rough in the previous year were more likely to report mental health problems than those who had not slept rough. Given the additional pressures of living on the streets it is not difficult to understand why.

Some people felt that homelessness had adversely affected their mental health. However, it is important to remember that all sorts of other problems and difficulties go hand in hand with homelessness and that people's reported mental health problems may be a reaction to these as well as to being homeless. For example, most single homeless people were unemployed and on very low incomes (Anderson et al.1993). The anxieties and depression of some homeless people might, therefore, be just as much to do with these problems as with the lack of a home.

A high proportion of single homeless people who reported mental health problems also reported heavy drinking. This applied to almost a third of those in hostels and B&Bs and almost half of those sleeping rough. This is much higher than expected – 10 per cent of the general population, according to the *Health of the Nation* (DoH 1993), are thought to suffer from both psychiatric and alcohol problems. In addition, many of the reasons single homeless people gave for leaving their last home were stressful events. For example, relationship breakdown was one of the commonest reasons given for leaving home (Anderson *et al.* 1993). Given that a strong association is known to exist between marital breakdown and mental illness (Dominian 1991), those who experience homelessness in addition to the breakdown of a relationship are at even greater risk of mental health problems. Furthermore, many single homeless people had stayed in institutions at some time in their lives. Almost a half of hostel and B&B residents, and seven out of ten people sleeping rough, had been in at least one form of institution, including a children's home, psychiatric hospital, alcohol or drug unit, prison and a young offenders' institution (Table 9.6). In other words, homelessness in itself may not *cause* mental health problems but it may be related to, or a consequence of, a stressful previous life event which may in turn exacerbate, or eventually trigger, mental health problems.

Many single homeless people who reported 'depression, anxiety or nerves' appeared to have had a longer-term psychiatric history. The survey found that one in four of those who reported mental health problems had been in a psychiatric hospital at some time in

Table 9.6 Percentage of people who had ever stayed in an institution

	Hostels & B&Bs (%)	Day centres (%)	Soup runs (%)
Children's home	15	24	24
Foster parents	10	9	12
General hospital for over 3 months	10	22	20
Psychiatric hospital	12	20	17
Alcohol unit	7	18	14
Drugs unit	3	4	4
Young offenders' institution	9	18	21
Prison or remand centre	25	49	46
At least one of the above	47	73	68
(Base)	(1,267)	(345)	(152)

Source: Anderson *et al.* (1993) *Single Homeless People*, London: HMSO. Own analysis

their lives. The relationship between homelessness, mental illness and discharge from psychiatric hospital is a complicated one and it is not possible to trace people's housing or psychiatric histories from this study. However, another important finding to emerge from this study was that only a minority (1 per cent) of single homeless people had been discharged from psychiatric hospital *directly* into hostel or B&B accommodation, or were sleeping rough immediately following discharge from a psychiatric hospital (1 per cent). These findings suggest, therefore, that the important issue is less to do with the outcome of immediate discharge from psychiatric hospital, whether that is through the closure of long-stay psychiatric hospitals or discharge from an acute admission, but of adequate long-term care in the community (see Craig and Timms 1992).

Furthermore, a high proportion of homeless people who had stayed in a psychiatric hospital had been in another institution during some time in their lives. In particular, many had also been in prison or a remand centre – one in four people in hostels and B&Bs, and six out of ten people sleeping rough, who had been in a psychiatric hospital had also been in prison or a remand centre. These findings suggest that many single homeless people are trapped in a 'revolving door' of homelessness, crime and mental illness. This is an important finding because, although the *Health of the Nation* (DoH 1993) recognises 'mentally disordered offenders' (*sic*) as a vulnerable group and recommends that they should be diverted from the criminal justice system, there is no mention of the contribution that stable accommodation might make in this process.

One in ten people in hostels and B&Bs who reported mental health problems said that this caused them difficulties in finding or keeping accommodation. This suggests that the mental health of some single homeless people may well be contributing towards their homelessness. Very little is known about the problems which people with mental health problems face in gaining access to housing. Kay and Legg (1986) found, however, that people with mental health problems experienced difficulties in understanding how the housing system worked and in gaining access to the services and support they needed. Although mental illness is one of the categories under which a homeless person may be accepted by a local authority as being in priority need, mental illness encompasses a range of conditions, and assessing a person's mental health is known to be problematic for housing officers (Evans and Duncan 1988).

Less than a third of single homeless people with mental health problems were receiving treatment – in other words, two-thirds of those with mental health problems were not being treated. People who had previously been in a psychiatric hospital were more likely to be receiving treatment for their mental health problems than those who had never been in a psychiatric hospital; even so, half this group were not receiving treatment. The perception of the psychiatric teams involved in the London Homeless Mentally Ill Initiative was that one of the problems in providing a service to homeless mentally ill people was keeping in contact with them largely because of problems in finding them permanent supported accommodation (House of Commons Health Committee 1994).

HEAVY DRINKING OR ALCOHOL-RELATED PROBLEMS

A high proportion of single homeless people reported heavy drinking or alcohol-related health problems; this applied to a third of people sleeping rough and one in ten people in hostels and B&Bs (Anderson *et al.* 1993). A strict comparison with the general population using the British Household Panel Survey data was not possible. However, the first of a series of annual health surveys classified 9 per cent of the general population as 'problem drinkers' (White *et al.* 1993), almost the same proportion as reported by people in hostels and B&Bs. Comparison with the data from this health survey suggests, therefore, that alcohol is perhaps more of a problem among people sleeping rough than among people in hostels. However, this may be due to the fact that many hostels do not accept people with alcohol problems or allow alcohol on their premises, and in this way people with alcohol problems are often excluded from hostels and may consequently end up sleeping rough.

A quarter of people in hostels and B&Bs and two-fifths of day-centre users who reported heavy drinking said that this health problem had caused them difficulties in finding or keeping accommodation. However, only a third of the people in hostels and B&Bs, and even fewer people sleeping rough, were receiving treatment for their heavy drinking. Although not everyone with alcohol-related problems may require treatment, many homeless people with alcohol-related problems had negative feelings about their health, and this suggests that more may have needed treatment than were receiving it. Furthermore, a very high proportion of those who reported heavy drinking, particularly those sleeping rough, had additional health problems (Table 9.7), and compared to the sample overall, single homeless people with alcohol problems had a higher risk of having other health problems. Vredevoe *et al.* (1992) showed that alcohol abuse among homeless people was an important risk factor for a number of health problems.

Overall, 7 per cent of people in hostels and B&Bs had been in an alcohol unit and at least twice as many sleeping rough had done so (Anderson *et al.* 1993). The proportion who had been in an alcohol unit was much higher among those who reported heavy drinking – almost two out of five had been in an alcohol unit. This is an important finding for two reasons: first, it suggests that heavy drinking was a recurring problem for two-fifths of those who reported it at the time

Table 9.7 Percentage of people reporting heavy drinking who had other health problems

Health problems	Hostels & B&Bs (%)	Day centres (%)	Soup runs (%)
No (other) health problems	11	11	7
One other health problem	17	16	11
More than one other health problem	72	74	83
Total	100	100	100
(Base)	(163)	(116)	(47)

Source: Single Homeless People Survey data (1991). Own analysis

of the survey; and second, it shows that alcohol units are a service used by a high proportion of single homeless people with alcohol problems. Any changes to the level of service provision are, therefore, likely to have a significant impact on homeless people.

ACCESS TO HEALTH CARE AND SUPPORT IN ACCOMMODATION

The *Patient's Charter* makes clear that every citizen has the right to be registered with a doctor. General practitioners hold the key to a range of primary health services and as such the problems of single homeless people registering with a doctor have been a main area of concern (Bayliss and Logan 1987; Stern *et al.* 1989). The survey of single homeless people found that 80 per cent of people in hostels and B&Bs, and 61 per cent of people using day centres, were registered with a doctor. The majority of single homeless people also said they knew of a medical centre or doctor to whom they could go if they felt unwell (Table 9.8).

Anderson *et al.* (1993) reported that more single homeless people knew of a doctor to whom they could go if feeling unwell, than were registered with a doctor. This was also the general impression given by single homeless people who took part in the group discussions. Greater use appeared to be made of medical facilities provided specifically for single homeless people in hostels or at day centres, or special health-care services, than of mainstream services. Some people, notably those who were younger, said they relied on hostel staff to call out a doctor if they were unwell. Some people mentioned how they varied which service they used depending on where they were staying. This varied use of health services has implications for the

Table 9.8 Percentage registered with a doctor or who knew of one to to go to for medical help

	Hostels & B&Bs (%)	Day centres (%)	Soup runs (%)
Registered with a doctor	80	61	NA
Knew of a doctor to whom they could go	90	85	78
(Base)	(1,278)	(351)	(155)

Source: Anderson *et al.* (1993) *Single Homeless People*, London: HMSO. Own analysis

planning of health-care services for single homeless people and for the effective delivery of those services.

Although the majority of single homeless people had access to primary health care, there were some people for whom this did not apply. Registering with a doctor was not considered by everyone to be problem-free; some homeless people felt they were discriminated against because they were homeless. People sleeping rough were less likely to have access to primary health care than people in hostels and B&Bs. People sleeping rough do not have an address and are, therefore, more likely to have problems in getting registered with a doctor because of this.

Being without a permanent home may mean frequent moves from one place to another. If the change of accommodation also involves moving to a different area this may have repercussions on access to primary health care. The survey found that people in hostels and B&Bs who had moved from their home city were less likely to be registered with a doctor, or to know of one to whom they could go, than those who were still living in the city in which they considered their last home to be. The task of having to register with a new doctor may be a daunting one for homeless people who are unfamiliar with the area to which they have moved, or uncertain as to how long they may be staying in the area.

The length of time that people had been homeless had little effect on whether they had access to health care, with the exception of people aged under twenty-five. The longer that they had been homeless, the *more* likely they were to know of a doctor to whom they could go if feeling unwell. This suggests that young people recently homeless may be less aware of the services and networks available to them than young people who had been homeless for longer. Similarly, the longer that young people had been in their hostel or B&B, the more likely they were to be registered with a doctor and to know of one to whom they could go if unwell. This may reflect the stability provided through longer-term stays in hostels and the efforts of hostel and resettlement staff in providing information about, and encouraging the use of, health facilities.

Despite the fact that the majority of single homeless people were registered with a doctor, Anderson *et al.* (1993) reported that many single homeless people were not receiving treatment for their health problems. Being registered with a doctor or knowing of one to go to does not necessarily imply that the service will be used. Even though treatment may be available, some homeless people may not be able to receive it. On the other hand, there were some homeless people who were not registered with a doctor but whose health problems were being treated. These findings suggest that registration rates should be treated with caution when used to monitor access to health care – they only tell part of the story and do not necessarily tell us much about usage of health-care services. This issue is examined in more detail in Pleace and Quilgars (this volume).

CONCLUSION

In recent years there has been growing concern about the health of single homeless people, although evidence to date has tended to come from small-scale or local studies. However, the findings in this chapter are based on the first national survey of single homeless people to be carried out since the late 1970s and as such provide an important contemporary source of information about the health of single homeless people.

The physical and mental health of single homeless people was found to be considerably worse than that of the general population. While it is difficult to know the direction of cause and effect between homelessness and poor health, the findings in this chapter nevertheless confirm that there is a strong relationship between the two. Many of the health problems that were particularly prevalent among single homeless people, such as chest, skin and musculoskeletal problems, were those that could conceivably be caused or made worse by sleeping rough. Mental health problems were experienced by many more single homeless people, especially those sleeping rough, than the general population. Although the causes for this are unclear, the findings suggest that there is a relationship between homelessness and mental health problems. Many single homeless people came from difficult backgrounds, were unemployed, on low incomes and had alcohol problems. Even if homelessness is not directly to blame for their mental health problems, the existence of other related problems, together with being homeless, makes it hardly surprising that so many did report feelings of depression, anxiety and nerves. Furthermore, many of those who reported mental health problems had a previous psychiatric history which suggests a more complicated relationship with homelessness.

People sleeping rough, who are experiencing the extreme end of the homelessness spectrum, were found to suffer the worst health of all. Other evidence suggests that those people sleeping rough who have alcohol and mental health problems and who have been homeless for a long time, are those for whom it is most difficult to find appropriate accommodation (Randall and Brown 1993). One of the most important findings from this study is that many single homeless people were suffering from multiple health problems. In many cases the combination of health problems, such as fits, mental illness and alcohol, could represent a serious risk to their well-being and safety. None of those interviewed in the survey had, however, been accepted by a local authority as vulnerable and in priority need for housing despite their poor health. Furthermore, the majority of those with health problems and particularly those with multiple problems said that they would require support in accommodation, and for many this included a range of different types of support. This suggests that there are a considerable number of vulnerable single people falling through the gaps of the homelessness legislation and community care provision. Greater attention needs to be drawn to the holistic needs of single homeless people to ensure that their health, housing and community care needs are appropriately met. This requires, as recommended by the Faculty of Public Health report (Connelly *et al.* 1992), greater liaison and collaboration between all sectors to ensure that the multiple needs of single homeless people are met. At the end of the day the health of single homeless people is as much the responsibility of housing, community care, employment and social security policies as it is for health policy.

NOTES

1 This chapter is an edited version of Bines (1994). The original contains extensive qualitative material and some additional tables. The British Household Panel Study (BHPS) data used in this paper were made available through the ESRC Data Archive. The data were originally collected by the ESRC Research Centre on Micro-social Change at the University of Essex. Neither the original collectors of the data nor the Archive bear any responsibility for the analyses or interpretations presented here.
2 Single homeless people were drawn from three different representative samples. These included a sample of people staying in hostels, night shelters and B&B hotels providing accommodation for single homeless people; and two samples of people sleeping rough (defined as having slept rough on at least one night out of the previous seven) who were using either day centres or soup runs for single homeless people.
    The survey of people in temporary accommodation was carried out in ten local authority case-study areas and the surveys of people sleeping rough were carried out in five of the local authority case-study areas. The case-study areas included five local authorities in London and five

outside London. These were selected using three different data sources: the homelessness returns made by local authorities to the Department of the Environment; the 1981 Census data on persons living in hostels and lodging houses; and for London, the *London Hostel Directory 1990*. Local authorities that had a high score on both indices (or on all three indices for London) were selected.

3   Two British studies which have compared the health of homeless people to the general population are known to the author; Shanks (1988) examined the morbidity of homeless people in Manchester and used the National Morbidity Survey as a comparison; Victor (1992) compared the health status of the temporarily homeless population of the North West Thames region and made comparisons with regional residents. An American study, Vredevoe *et al.* (1992), compared the health of homeless people in Los Angeles with data on non-homeless people taken from the 1985 National Ambulatory Medical Care Survey.

4   This was calculated by applying the age- and gender-specific rates for each of the health problems in the standard population (taken from the BHPS) to the number of single homeless people in each of the age and gender groups. An expected number of single homeless people with each of the health problems was then obtained (E). The expected figure was then compared to the actual or observed number (O) of single homeless people reporting the health problem (O/E). This was multiplied by 100 to obtain a ratio.

5   The findings relating to 'heart problems' should be treated with some caution since the definitions used in the two surveys were slightly different. Single homeless people were asked about 'heart problems' whereas the general population was asked about 'heart/blood or circulation problems'. There is, therefore, the possibility that single homeless people under-reported this type of health problem because of the omission of blood pressure or circulation problems from the question.

6   Strictly comparable figures are not possible for the general population. However, the Health Service Indicators show that the national average hospitalisation rate for mental illness admissions per 1,000 district residents in 1990/91 was 4.61 and this figure only changed marginally in subsequent years.

Chapter 10

Health, homelessness and access to health care services in London

Nicholas Pleace and Deborah Quilgars

This chapter considers the relationships between health status and homelessness, drawing particularly on research undertaken by the authors for the King's Fund in London during 1995.[1] The chapter begins by considering what the associations between homelessness and poor health actually mean and moves on to argue that the high prevalence of health problems experienced by homeless people is only one element of the problem. Within London, the issue is not simply that homeless people have poor health status, but also that they frequently cannot get adequate access to health services. The chapter then moves on to argue that improving access to health services is not an answer to the poor health of homeless people, and it is only by reducing levels of homelessness that the issue can be adequately addressed.

HEALTH AND HOMELESSNESS

The extensive literature on health and homelessness in the United Kingdom and the rest of the industrialised world tells a very similar story. Homelessness is very bad for your health, especially if you are someone who spends time sleeping on the street. A street homeless person in New York, Japan or London is much more likely than the general population of those countries to catch tuberculosis (Concato and Rom 1994; Yamanaka *et al.* 1994; Citron *et al.* 1995). If one is homeless in an advanced industrialised nation, there is also a much higher chance that one will have a mental health problem than members of the general population (Craig and Timms 1992; Cohen and Thompson 1992; Geddes *et al.* 1994). Bines's work reported in this volume (Chapter 9) demonstrates the disproportionate prevalence of health problems among single homeless people in England.

Much of the literature hammers these lessons home, some of it with echoes of the zeal with which Victorian reformers condemned the conditions in which the poor had to exist. The situation which research has found has perhaps meant that the existing literature is often heavy with moral outrage, but light on analysis. The Royal College of Physicians (1994) recently began to protest about the standard of some studies of health and homelessness. They pointed to an absence of any comparison between the health of homeless people and other sections of the population with similar characteristics. The bias of some research, which made statements about the prevalence of health problems among all homeless people by looking only at the health of homeless people who used health services, was also noted.

On one level, it could be argued that relatively poor academic standards in some studies of health and homelessness are not terribly important. These studies, while perhaps not always rigorous, are nevertheless consistently demonstrating a high prevalence of health problems among homeless people. However, to follow this argument avoids discussion of a shortcoming within much of what has been written on health and homelessness, which is the often implicit assumption that homelessness *causes* ill health.

There are a number of problems with this assumption. The causes of ill health are complex and affect different people in different ways. Many factors represent a *risk* to health, but the fact that they are present or absent does not always mean that someone will or will not become unwell. It is known that smoking, saturated fat, lack of exercise and stress are all bad for us, but it would be quite wrong to suggest that eliminating these factors from our lives would always mean that we would not become unwell. Equally, we know that not everyone who smokes, drinks too much or eats too many of the wrong things will develop health problems because of these activities. Although healthier living means a better chance of an active and long life, it does not guarantee it. A genetic disposition to certain diseases, infectious disease or inherited characteristics leading to health problems also cannot necessarily be countered by a healthier lifestyle. Our understanding of what causes ill health, such as recent indications about the role of stress levels in all aspects of health, also changes over time (Taylor and Bloor 1994).

Becoming homeless does not *guarantee* poor health. Rather, being homeless can mean an increased risk that someone will develop health problems. Living in overcrowded and insanitary conditions, as many homeless people do, means that they are at an increased risk of getting infectious diseases, and the stress associated with what is a horrendous situation probably has a role in the prevalence of mental health problems among homeless people. All the problems associated with poverty also increase the risks to health: poor living conditions, poor diet, exposure to damp and cold and so forth. Homeless people also tend to be at greater physical risk from assault or accidents (the latter through cramped living conditions). Homelessness, then, represents an increased risk to health, and like other risks to health, it will not always cause health problems in the individuals and families who experience it.

Once the factors within homelessness that lead to risks of health problems developing are unpicked, it quickly becomes apparent that few of them are unique to homeless people as a group. Any relatively economically deprived section of the population is exposed to similar and often identical risks to health. Victor (1992) compared the health of homeless people in temporary accommodation across several central London boroughs with that of the housed population (many of whom lived in social housing) and found that the high prevalence of acute illness and longstanding limiting illness was very *similar* in the housed and homeless populations. Lissauer *et al.* (1993) found that homeless children admitted to a central London hospital had fewer pronounced health problems than housed children, although three homeless children died after admission, whereas none of the housed children did. These studies indicated that although single homeless people and homeless families in central London had poor health status, their situation was not unique. The problem of relatively poor health status is one faced by every socioeconomically deprived group within the population.

Although the risks to health experienced by many homeless people are not exceptional, one group does face a range of risk factors that are not experienced by any other element of the population – people sleeping rough. All homeless people are by definition very badly accommodated, but this group spends time sleeping outside, exposed to danger from assault, and to the weather. The work of Anderson *et al.* (1993) and Bines (1994; this volume) has indicated that the health status of people sleeping rough is worse than that of other single homeless people. Work among street homeless people in the United States has had similar findings (Zolopa *et al.* 1994; Concato and Rom 1994). However, with the notable exception of people sleeping rough, homelessness does not consistently constitute a unique risk to health.

Another problem exists with the assumption in some research that homelessness causes poor health status. This problem is in the failure of some research to recognise the possible relationships between cause and effect. The best example of this comes from the debate around homelessness and mental health problems in the United States. In the mid-1980s, research appeared that argued that the rise in street homelessness was caused by the closure of state mental hospitals. Homeless people were increasing in number because people with a mental health problem were being discharged from long-stay hospitals, could not cope and ended up on skid row (Basuk 1984). More recently, research began to appear that disputed this, arguing that becoming a street homeless person in the United States drove individuals who were previously healthy into developing a mental health problem (Winkleby and White 1992; Cohen and Thompson 1992). Both these arguments, which are meant to contradict each other, are probably at least partially right.

The relationship between the extent to which becoming homeless causes health status to deteriorate and the extent to which people may become homeless because they have poor health status is not properly understood. It is, almost certainly, the case that becoming homeless causes mental health to deteriorate; this is common sense, anyone living in awful conditions or who may have escaped violence or abuse is hardly likely to be in good mental health. It is also known that most of the homeless people who have mental health problems in the United Kingdom are *not* people from long-stay hospitals that have closed (Craig and Timms 1992). On the other hand, the more sophisticated analyses of single homelessness (Dant and Deacon 1989; Vincent *et al.* 1995; Caton 1990) at least hint at a potential role for mental health problems in increasing the risk of homelessness, because the socio-economic forces that cause homelessness seem to affect the most vulnerable groups within society disproportionately.

Homelessness does not represent a cause of poor health, but an increased risk to health. The risks to health are in most instances not unique, although there is evidence that people sleeping rough experience a level of risk to their health beyond that found in any other section of the population. The poor health status of at least some homeless people may pre-date their homelessness and may even be a factor that exacerbated their chances of becoming homeless in the first place.

It could be argued that these qualifications are merely academic. The bottom line is still that homeless people have poor health and the problem is as simple as that. However, this is the point at which the real problem with many existing studies arises. Not only do these studies, by not considering the detail properly, misrepresent the relationship between poor health and homelessness, they quite often miss or only skirt around the real difference between homeless people and other socio-economically deprived sections of the population when it comes to health. While a person living on benefit in social housing, who experiences similar risks to health to many homeless people, may not enjoy the same quality of access to health services as someone from the middle class (Black *et al.* 1992), their access to health services is still likely to be a lot better than that of a homeless person. The main impact, the unique impact, of homelessness on health in the United Kingdom is that it restricts or even prevents access to health services.

ACCESS TO THE NHS FOR HOMELESS PEOPLE IN LONDON

Registration with a GP is the main means by which people in the United Kingdom receive medical services. Those services that are not provided by the GP directly are arranged and accessed by their referrals. Without access to a GP, one not only cannot receive basic medical care, but also referral to more specialist services can become very difficult. Two forms of registration exist at the time of writing. Permanent registration gives someone full access to a GP. Temporary registration (originally designed for travelling workers and people on holiday) gives access to a GP, but one's medical records are not transferred and a medical card is not issued. People can also be treated by GPs under emergency treatment rules for twenty-four hours.

Homeless people are disadvantaged by this system in several ways. GPs receive finance on the basis of the number of registered patients that they have. A permanently registered patient who moves before the end of a financial year takes the money that is associated with her or him to a new area. In contrast, if the patient is temporarily registered, a GP can guarantee income from that person for up to nine months. As throughout the rest of the NHS, GPs have to be increasingly aware of financial considerations. Homeless people tend to move around a lot. People sleeping rough and single homeless people may move between areas, not necessarily through choice, but to try to find services. Statutorily homeless people, housed under the 1985 Act, could be moved by a local authority to temporary accommodation before they are finally rehoused and, under the pending legislative changes in the 1996 Housing Act, they could be in temporary accommodation for up to two years. Permanently registering a family or individual that may only be in an area for a few weeks or months makes no sense to a GP in budgetary terms, yet many homeless people fall into this category (Fisher and Collins 1993). Within London, this problem is especially acute, since GP patches are often very small because the population is so dense. Homeless people moving a few miles could easily pass through more than one GP's patch. Since medical records are not transferred when someone is temporarily registered, the continuity of care that the NHS provides through the registration system is frequently not available to homeless people. Temporary registration also means that someone has no medical card with which to access some health services.

GPs can also refuse to take people onto their lists. Registration can be refused unless the local Health Authority (previously the Family Health Services Authority) obliges them to take someone onto their lists for up to three months. Inner-city GPs can fear being 'swamped' by homeless people if they register a few individuals, and often view homeless people as difficult or challenging individuals who would affect them and their other patients. The popular conception of homeless people as disruptive and drug- or alcohol-dependent still permeates society. Some commentators have also suggested that the very poor health status of some homeless people makes them relatively expensive to register and that this may be a disincentive when budgets are very tight, though no research has yet confirmed this assertion (Fisher and Collins 1993). Registration systems may also work against homeless people, since many GPs' systems assume that anyone who wishes to use their services should have a permanent address in order to register permanently, something that homeless people by definition do not have.

In addition to the administrative, budgetary and prejudicial barriers to registration, there are also other difficulties that have to be overcome. Some homeless people can be individuals who are socially marginalised or who lack the skills with which to deal with bureaucracy or express themselves. Low educational levels may make it difficult for homeless people to advance their case, particularly if faced with a hostile receptionist or health professional. Within London, homeless people are also competing with the rest of the population for health services that are increasingly under pressure in trying to meet the various demands placed upon them.

Several studies within London have indicated that registration rates among homeless people are poor. Research into the high use of hospital accident and emergency services (A&E) by homeless people has often assumed that this reflected poor registration levels (HVA and GMSC 1988; Victor *et al.* 1989; Scheuer *et al.* 1991). This may be partially true, although other studies have found high registration rates among homeless people existing alongside high use of A&E, which may mean that high use of A&E simply reflects the poor health status of many homeless people (Victor 1992). Alternatively, homeless people may be registered, but have moved from the area where their GP is based. Two detailed studies by Hinton (1992 and 1994) in London have demonstrated low registration levels (60 per cent registered, compared with 98–99 per cent of the general population) among people sleeping rough and lower registration rates among single homeless people than the general population. People sleeping rough in London interviewed for the King's Fund research in 1995 confirmed that it was often difficult to get access to GPs, especially if one had a drug or alcohol dependency: 'You can't register with a doctor. The only ones you can see is either in the hospital, or here, or Great Chapel Street [medical centre for homeless people]' (homeless man in his late teens in London, 1995).

Within hospitals in London, the attitudes of staff towards homeless people and service provision for homeless people have sometimes been criticised. Homeless people can be viewed by hospital staff in A&E departments as 'inappropriate attenders', because they have health-care needs that could be addressed by a GP. Negative staff attitudes can also be linked to the high levels of dependence on drugs and alcohol among some groups of homeless people and a feeling that their health problems are to some extent self-inflicted. There is some evidence that single homeless people can be kept waiting longer than some patients, that received treatment can be cursory and that follow-up and discharge arrangements are often inadequate (Martin *et al.* 1992; Hinton 1994; Pleace and Quilgars 1996).

Evidence on the use of inpatient services by homeless people is very limited, both within London and elsewhere. One comparative study looking at the admission of homeless and housed children found that the decision to admit was often related to homelessness itself. The homeless children admitted into one London hospital had generally less severe illness than the housed children, but decisions to admit were taken because social factors (namely homelessness) were thought to undermine the chance of recovery if the children were not admitted (Lissauer *et al.* 1993). Given what is known about problems with access to GP services and A&E services, it is perhaps not unreasonable to surmise that access to inpatient services is problematic for homeless people, because the main routes into a hospital bed are themselves difficult for homeless people to use.

Much has been written about the generally poor state of mental health services within the capital and throughout the United Kingdom as a whole (Audit Commission 1994). Access to mental health services for homeless people can be difficult for many of the same reasons that access to other health services is poor, but there is the added problem that these services are often restricted and under extreme pressure. While improvements are being sought, service intervention often only comes at the point at which someone is in crisis, and provision to prevent deterioration and for people who are recovering from severe mental illness is generally restricted. Homeless people are therefore disadvantaged by being homeless and by being in competition with everyone else who needs assistance from inadequate services. For those homeless people who are dependent on drugs or alcohol and who have a mental health problem, a particular difficulty exists, which is the low number of services for homeless people with both a dependency and a mental health problem in London (Pleace and Quilgars 1996).

A LIMITED RESPONSE

Across central London there is an extensive range of medical services available solely or mainly for homeless people. Provision such as Great Chapel Street Medical Centre, the specialist outreach teams provided under the Homeless Mentally Ill Initiative (funded by the Department of Health) and the primary care teams and services provided within day centres, all fulfil a vital role in delivering health care to homeless people. Evidence of the need for these services is considerable; for example, in 1995 figures from the Great Chapel Street Medical Centre off Oxford Street showed it had seen 18,500 patients and undertaken 82,000 consultations over the previous fifteen years (Great Chapel Street 1995). Many health authorities in central London were also providing at least some services designed to improve access to health services for homeless people (Pleace and Quilgars 1996).

These responses, although undoubtedly valuable, did not address the underlying problem for homeless people in gaining access to health care in London. The difficulty stemmed not from the range or extent of adaptations to existing NHS provision in the capital or the availability of specialist services designed solely for homeless people, although both could have been improved. Rather, the root of the problem was homelessness itself.

Clearly, no matter how well designed and operated health services for homeless people are, they will not be able in themselves to address the problem of poor health status among homeless people. Of course, ending homelessness will not solve the problem of poor health status because, although homeless people will (probably) experience a reduction in the number or level of risk factors to their health, they will still be living with similar or perhaps equivalent levels of risk when their homelessness ceases. Formerly homeless people tend to live in the social rented or private rented sectors, quite often in housing that is not of a very high standard, they find it difficult to find work and may spend much or all their lives on benefit. In short, people who have been homeless are frequently moving from a (sometimes extreme) position of socio-economic disadvantage into another position of socio-economic disadvantage, which means the risks to their health are still greater than those faced by the general population (Dant and Deacon 1989; Black *et al.* 1992; Pleace 1995, and this volume; Vincent *et al.* 1995).

However, although ending homelessness will not necessarily greatly reduce the risks to a homeless person's health, there are three basic reasons why an attempt should be made to reduce greatly the levels of homelessness in society in order to meet the health-care needs of homeless people. First, any improvement is better than nothing. Whereas the level of accommodation, financial support and other assistance that can be made available to homeless people will not lift them out of relative poverty, the risks to their health will almost certainly lessen even if the accommodation and benefits they receive are merely adequate. Second, the current policy of concerning ourselves with the health of homeless people, but not with their homelessness, is at least partially illogical. While it can be argued that the NHS routinely delivers services to people who are at disproportionate risk of health problems, there is a point at which it becomes illogical to do this, because any intervention is unlikely to have any effect. The situation in which some homeless people, especially people sleeping rough, find themselves, can overwhelm any attempt at treatment.

Third, the provision of an address is the only way around the problem of access to health services. The NHS is designed to function on a geographical basis, it can cope with people moving, but like community care as a whole, it needs housing and permanent addresses as a means to administer the delivery of services. The basic point of access to NHS services is registration with a GP and permanent registration generally requires an address.

There is another aspect to the findings of the authors' recent research. London, one of the major cities in the world, has had services organised for the sizeable homeless population within the city for many years. The problem of poor health status has persisted among homeless people, despite a developed health-service response, high levels of voluntary service provision and individual service developments by individual boroughs. To a considerable extent, this situation could be viewed as one in which one possible policy response – adapting the NHS to accommodate homeless people and the provision of specialised services to homeless people – although it has done a great deal for the homeless population in London, has been tried and has failed. Addressing homelessness, which is admittedly sometimes more complex than simply making affordable homes available, especially for single homeless people, may now be the only means left by which the poor health of homeless people can itself be addressed.

NOTES

1   Full details of the research can be found in Pleace and Quilgars (1996).

Chapter 11

Rehousing single homeless people

Nicholas Pleace

The focus of this chapter is on the rehousing of single homeless people accepted under the 1985 Housing Act as statutorily homeless (Pleace *et al.* this volume; Lowe, this volume). While the causes of single homelessness and the impact that it can have on an individual have been researched extensively, it is only in recent years that attention has been brought to bear on what happens to single homeless people after they are rehoused. The chapter begins with a brief discussion of how the problems that can arise for single homeless people when they are rehoused were gradually recognised. It then moves on to discuss the results of research undertaken by the author in 1994, and concludes by arguing that while the needs of formerly single homeless people for services in addition to housing are increasingly recognised, service provision is currently inadequate.

REHOUSING TO RESETTLEMENT

The first 'explanation' of single homelessness that emerged was simply that single homeless people chose homelessness as a lifestyle, refusing both responsibility and work. This view of single homelessness was unchallenged until the 1960s, when research appeared that made the first links between poor health, mental health problems, alcohol dependency and homelessness.

The research that linked single homelessness to poor health represented the first attempt to understand homelessness systematically. The argument that poor health causes homelessness is still advanced by some academics today, although it is now largely found within the American literature on street and shelter homelessness. The basic theory is that single homeless people become homeless because they are relatively vulnerable and unable to function in society. In other words, those adults who are least capable of looking after themselves are those adults who become homeless. This may be because of a mental health problem that undermines a person's ability to work, maintain or form relationships or cope with the pressures of day-to-day living (Basuk 1984; Wolf 1990). Homeless people are not to 'blame' for their homelessness; rather, they are homeless because they are unable to cope within society. There is overwhelming evidence to suggest that single homeless people are much more likely than the general population to have poor physical health and mental health problems (Royal College of Physicians 1994; Barry *et al.* 1991; Bines 1994, and this volume).

However, on closer examination it soon became apparent that this argument was running into difficulties when it came to demonstrating cause and effect. If, for example, mental health problems are a cause of homelessness, why does almost everyone who develops a mental health problem in the United States or the United Kingdom *not* become homeless? In addition, the argument that illness leads to homelessness does not take account of the possibility of health problems developing because a previously healthy individual is exposed to many health risks when they become homeless (Snow and Anderson 1987; Cohen and Thompson 1992).

In response to the problems with the 'poor health causes homelessness' theory, a new argument developed that emphasised the structural causes of single homelessness. This approach was based on the view that housing supply and socio-economic changes cause homelessness. It was agreed that only some single homeless people had support needs, most did not, and only required adequate and affordable housing. A government report, *Single and Homeless*, completed by Drake *et al.* in 1982 was the most notable exponent of this view (Kemp, this volume). Most academics now accept that socio-economic factors have a important role in causing single homelessness (Bramley 1993; Anderson 1994).

However, while single homelessness was clearly caused by socio-economic factors, it was also clear that the arguments about health problems causing homelessness, while not robust, were drawing on significant data. Single homeless people do have more health problems than the general population, and some evidence suggested that people sleeping rough have the worst health problems of all (Bines, this volume).

This difficulty with the purely socio-economic argument led, in turn, to another set of arguments, which advanced the view that single homeless people were often (but not always) those who were *most vulnerable* to the socio-economic and housing supply factors that caused homelessness (Caton 1990). This is a much more rigorous argument than the first three, drawing heavily on our existing knowledge of the way in which post-industrial societies work. In effect, this approach argues that single homeless people represent something akin to an underclass of economically and socially marginalised people who are disproportionately characterised by being unskilled and having poor health status. When social housing provision in the United Kingdom, or the very cheap end of the private rented sector in the United States, becomes constricted, some of the most vulnerable individuals who would have lived in it become homeless. Equally, as the economies in industrial societies come under pressure and change, unskilled work is harder to find and access to adequate benefits may become more difficult, leading to increases in homeless. Of course, there are still problems with this argument, which does not explain why relatively few of the most marginalised people in society experience homelessness. It may be that another factor, perhaps individual experience, is also at work.

It has also become apparent that at least some single homeless people are alienated by the experiences that had made them homeless, or by the experience of homelessness itself. In the United Kingdom, the work of Dant and Deacon (1989) and Vincent *et al.* (1993) has shown that single homelessness among male hostel dwellers is often associated with an exclusion from employment, family relationships, friendships and sexual relationships along with an absence of possessions. In the United States, a similar phenomenon has been characterised as 'social dysfunction', an increasing inability to function within society associated with an increasing marginalisation from relationships and 'normal' life (Grigsby *et al.* 1990; Ziefert and Brown 1991). This form of alienation may have other effects, a lack of involvement with day-to-day living might mean that an individual has no idea how to run a flat, organise money or cook for themselves, so practical support may also be necessary, especially when someone has been homeless for a long time.

As understanding of single homelessness changes and, it is to be hoped, increases, it becomes apparent that the task of rehousing many single homeless people is far from simple. It is clearly illogical to try to meet the needs of single homeless people simply by providing them with an adequate and affordable home; there is a range of other needs that may need to be addressed:

1 *Housing need.* Housing must clearly be of a reasonable standard, affordable and secure. In addition, housing must be suitable for the particular needs of each single homeless person, which may sometimes require the use of specially designed or adapted homes.
2 *Support needs.* This includes medical needs and any need for personal care or support services, such as assistance with tasks associated with daily living, like cooking, dressing oneself or washing oneself, when one is unable to complete such tasks.
3 *Daily living skills.* Some single homeless people may not have had time or an opportunity to learn how to manage a flat or day-to-day living. This can apply particularly to young single homeless people who have left care or who left home suddenly. This is distinct from support needs, involving (for example) teaching someone how to cook for themselves because they are untrained rather than meeting a support need and cooking for them because they are unable to do it for themselves.
4 *Financial needs.* Homelessness is, of course, associated with relative poverty. Access to benefits for some single people who become homeless, particularly 16- and 17-year-olds, is restricted and some research has questioned the availability of the Social Fund for homeless people (Citizens' Advice Scotland, May 1994).
5 *Social needs.* Research suggests that homeless people may have a need for reintegration into society which resettlement services can address to some extent by the provision of some emotional support and practical assistance. In addition to possible alienation, there may also be problems around isolation and a lack of activity during the day that need to be addressed.

The remainder of this chapter discusses research undertaken in 1994 that examined the rehousing services of four local authority housing departments. The research was concerned both with the extent to which these different factors were important in effectively rehousing single homeless people and with the extent to which various agencies provided services which met these different needs.[1]

RESETTLEMENT

During 1994, interviews were conducted in four local authority housing departments and with a sample of the previously homeless single people they had housed under the 1985 Housing Act. Older people who were unable to manage living alone, people with learning difficulties, people with a mental health problem, disabled people, women escaping violence, vulnerable young people and people with other special needs, such as people with HIV/AIDS, were among those who could be accepted by these departments (DoE 1991). At the time of writing, acceptance by a local authority under the 1985 Act gives single homeless people priority access to permanent housing, which means that unlike other households seeking council or housing association accommodation they should not spend any time on the waiting list.

One authority was a London borough, another was a town on the south coast and the other two were major cities in the north of England. Between them, in 1993, these authorities housed 5,000 homeless households as vulnerable under the terms of the Act (about 70 per cent of which were single people) (Pleace *et al.* this volume) and controlled about 200,000 dwellings, which was around 5 per cent of the total council stock in England at the time. All the housing departments that agreed to take part in the study interpreted the code of guidance to the 1985 Housing Act relatively liberally and accepted higher than average numbers of single homeless people (Niner 1989; Butler *et al.* 1994).

Three of the housing departments had developed housing support and resettlement services designed to resettle single homeless people. These services mainly provided low-level support and helped formerly homeless people get into contact with social services and health services. The authority that had not made such provision had nevertheless developed an intensive housing management service for its temporary accommodation and had built social services care assessors into its homelessness acceptance procedures. The housing departments had developed these services because of their experience when rehousing single homeless people. It had become increasingly apparent that simply providing accommodation was not enough and that support was needed to counteract the tendency of many formerly homeless individuals being unable to manage in their new homes and returning to homelessness.

Meeting housing needs

The provision of suitable housing was one of the main difficulties that the housing departments faced. The demand on council housing in their areas meant that many single homeless people had to wait several months in unsuitable temporary accommodation and, when stock became available, its design and location were not always appropriate.

The problems began within some temporary accommodation. In three areas, there was quite high dependence on council-run hostels. Although the physical conditions in these hostels, which were very basic, were not criticised by the single homeless people living within them, the hostels were often thought, by both staff and residents, to be unsafe environments. Disorder and crime, particularly in all-male hostels, combined with a high incidence of mental health problems and drug and alcohol addiction within a relatively vulnerable group of residents to create a sometimes volatile mixture: 'It can create management hell . . . we've had people chucking themselves out of the windows here, we've had people setting fire to the skip outside, we've had people stabbing people, we've had drug dealing, we've had everything' (manager of a mixed hostel run by a London borough).

In addition to trying to keep the hostels as safe environments, housing staff had to deal with sometimes highly distressed homeless people who might undertake self-harming actions or cause widespread disruption and sometimes physical damage to the buildings.

Within temporary housing, which the housing department on the south coast made heavy use of, management problems of a similar sort had occurred, particularly when individuals with mental health problems or who were vulnerable in another way either caused disruption or were the targets of abuse. Difficulties could be especially pronounced if the department had to house several young homeless men in the same house. In addition, conditions within the temporary accommodation housing provided or arranged by all four housing departments could sometimes be poor.

Major problems also existed with regard to the provision of suitable permanent accommodation within the local authorities' own stock. The only housing available was usually in the form of unfurnished flats in low- or high-rise blocks. Again, there were concerns about crime in many areas in which this housing was situated and some disabled formerly homeless people felt very unsafe in their homes: 'I was out one day, twenty minutes, went to the shop down the road there. When I come back, no windows, they broke the lot' (formerly homeless man in his 60s, northern city).

The design and location of properties would be thought to affect whether or not a formerly homeless person could settle within them.

However, the research could not really test this idea, because the housing departments had very little choice available and would simply try to place homeless people in the most suitable accommodation they could find. This was held by many of the staff interviewed as an inadequate response and one that made failure more likely. The rehousing of homeless people with a mental health problem in noisy and disruptive buildings, the inappropriate rehousing of women escaping violence on estates with very high crime rates, and the placement of young people and others miles away from friends, family and other support networks were all given as examples of the problems the restricted range of available stock had generated: 'There is a shortage of appropriate accommodation ... so when we come to house single vulnerable people our options are limited, not because we do not recognise the level of need, but because we can only allocate what we have' (senior member of housing staff, southern town).

Finally, the attitude of neighbours could also be a problem. Existing tenants often associated young people with crime and displayed bigotry against people from certain groups in society. There was also intolerance directed against people with a mental health problem, especially if they were disruptive in some way.

Meeting support needs

All the housing departments had drawn on their experiences over the last decade or more to establish services to try to meet the support needs of the single homeless people that they rehoused. As noted above, repeated experience of formerly homeless single people being unable to manage when they were simply provided with a flat had led to the development of the in-house housing support worker teams in three authorities and the integration of social services into assessment procedures in the southern town.

Many management problems on estates and within temporary accommodation were very strongly associated in the view of housing management staff with generally poor co-ordination between housing departments, social services and the health service. In essence, people who required support from health and social services were seen as not getting that support, and disruption, problems with neighbours, abandonment of accommodation and even self-harm resulted.

In three authorities, homeless people in temporary accommodation and formerly homeless people in permanent accommodation were being supported by key workers or housing support workers with a limited, or even non-existent, input from health or social services. In these areas, untrained housing management staff were, in effect, sometimes providing the *only* support that homeless and formerly homeless people were receiving, even when the individuals in question had very pronounced support needs. In the housing authority on the south coast, co-operation between housing and social services was quite developed at the point of assessment, but less developed after that, while co-ordination with health services was as poor as in the other areas.

> When we've made a referral to social services, it can be anything up to six weeks before you get an acknowledgement. In the meantime this individual is becoming more and more dependent on the resettlement service support and if they should be lucky enough to get a support worker from social services the input isn't a great deal, we don't feel anyway. They'll come and do an assessment of the individual, point out to the individual what they can actually offer and, invariably, are quite clear as to when they will withdraw, it's almost like 'you get your problems sorted out in the next two months because I will no longer be able to offer that', their case load is such that they don't have the time.
>
> (Housing Support Team manager, northern city)

The problems, both for single homeless people and for housing management staff acting on their behalf, in getting access to community care and health services were held to be caused by two factors. First, agencies other than housing were sometimes reluctant to take responsibility for homeless people, who, no matter how vulnerable or unwell they were, had in recent years fallen outside the direct priorities of health and social services. Second, and in the view of some housing management staff much more important, community care and health service commissioners and providers had insufficient resources to cope with the demands from homeless people as they were already struggling to meet very great demand from other sections of the population.

An absence of support, as earlier research had suggested, could mean that homeless people were unable to resettle and sometimes that they could not even stay for very long in temporary accommodation before returning to homelessness. Among those people who were rehoused, the absence of health and social services input, or access to services for only a relatively short time or on an infrequent basis, was sometimes leading to a poor quality of life, both for themselves and in some instances for their neighbours. High levels of stress were reported by housing staff with a resettlement role, and housing managers responsible for the estates on which some single homeless people were rehoused reported spending a lot of their time trying to arrange community care services for formerly homeless people who were in distress.

While they attempted to try to meet support needs among single homeless people, either through arranging community care services or through limited provision of low-level support, all the housing departments were very conscious of the limits placed on the extent of their 'welfare' role by government (DoE 1994c). Housing departments were expected to concentrate on housing management tasks, repairing properties and collecting the rent, and not to devote resources to the welfare of individual vulnerable tenants, who were the responsibility of health and social services. The housing departments themselves were organisations devoted to providing efficient housing management for the large sections of the population in their area who lived in the homes they provided, and were reluctant, at policy level, to move resources away from these core activities. These pressures, combined with a situation of general fiscal constraint within the housing departments, meant that they could not, and did not want to, provide substitute health or social services for the homeless people that they rehoused. Housing support workers and key workers could often only spend less than an hour every week with each single homeless person they were responsible for, caseloads for individual workers sometimes ranging between forty and eighty.

> We offer housing, we offer so much support, if a woman is having a bad day and wants to talk about it, she can talk about it, but don't take all day because there are other things to do. It's not that brutal, but we have to refer them to other agencies.
>
> (Worker, women's hostel, northern city)

Meeting needs for training in daily living skills

The housing support worker services for people in temporary or permanent housing and the key worker services within hostels had moved away from the provision of training in daily living skills, focusing instead on the more pressing difficulty of getting access to care and support services for single homeless people. This was seen by both staff and homeless people themselves as something of a problem when it came to the increasing number of young people that the authorities were accepting as homeless. Young people who had left care, or who had only just left home, were unlikely to have the skills necessary to run their own home.

> There isn't actually anything in here, no programme when some-one comes in and says we are going to have a meeting on how to sort out an electric bill. The kids that come in here, they are dead young and they are not going to have a clue. I mean I never even wrote a cheque out till Christmas and I was 25 at Christmas.
>
> (Formerly homeless woman, northern city)

MEETING FINANCIAL NEEDS

All the homeless people that the authorities accepted for rehousing were relatively poor, but particular problems existed for the 16- and 17-year-olds, who had very restricted access to benefits under government rules. The housing departments' housing management and housing support worker staff sought financial assistance for single homeless people from every conceivable source. All stored and redistributed any furniture left by vacating tenants, had links with any charities that could provide furniture or grants and used the key workers and housing support workers to explore the mazes of the benefits system on behalf of the single homeless people they housed. Nevertheless, little or no income could lead to abandonment of flats by formerly homeless 16- and 17-year-olds, and living at a subsistence level was commonplace among those formerly home-less people who were managing to stay in their flats: 'You tend to find that when they have been given a tenancy, and they've had to give it up fairly quickly for whatever reason and you go in there, all that's in the flat is a mattress, that's all they've had' (estate manager, northern city).

MEETING SOCIAL NEEDS

Within hostels, key workers were often acutely aware of the isolation that single homeless people had experienced and often took the view that this made them vulnerable to exploitation and abuse. Homeless people often formed very close relationships extremely quickly, and key workers reported that inappropriate, intense and one-sided relationships would sometimes form between themselves and the individuals to whom they were providing a service.

We had, I think, 400 women through here last year and there's probably only handful of them actually have friends. Which, well, most of us have friends, its like they don't know anyone, their friendships will be made in here and they're not real, it's amazing, people say oh, she's like my sister, within a day of meeting them in here. Nobody will come and see them and they've got no one to go and see, some of the young people want friends but they don't know how to choose friends or say no to people.

(Manager, women's hostel, northern city)

Once homeless people had been settled in permanent accommodation, the picture was more mixed. While some relied on the contact and support provided by their visits from housing support workers, most had formed their own social networks and were managing rather better than might be predicted from a review of the literature dealing with social exclusion and alienation among single homeless people. However, these individuals were people who had been relatively successful in the rehousing process, often managing in their own flat for several months.

DISCUSSION

Understanding the relative importance of the different elements of service provision in the rehousing of single homeless people was made rather difficult by the situation in which the local housing departments were operating. All the authorities had sold a lot of their better housing stock under the Right to Buy and were unable to replace it; co-ordination with other agencies was difficult because of financial constraints and other factors; and the resettlement services that were provided by the authorities were under very considerable strain. In short, it was not possible really to test the effectiveness or the importance of many types of service that might be beneficial in the rehousing of single homeless people because these services were often unavailable or available in only a limited or flawed form.

Having made this clear, the research did provide further evidence that these services are often necessary, that there were high levels of support need among single homeless people, and this clearly did make a difference when it came to rehousing them successfully. Social needs and requirements for training in daily living skills were not universally present, but were nevertheless a factor for significant numbers of the single homeless people that the authorities were rehousing. There was little difference between the view that housing staff took of the needs of homeless people and the views that they themselves expressed about their own needs. The similarity between the current academic understanding of single homelessness and the underlying ideas behind the design of the rehousing services the local authorities were providing was also very considerable.

It is also apparent that questions need to be asked as to why a section of society that clearly contains many very vulnerable individuals does not have proper access to the community care, social support, medical and housing services it requires, even when its members cease to be homeless and are 'permanently' rehoused by local authorities.

While it is important to examine the non-housing needs of single homeless people if services are to be designed that can effectively stop them from being homeless and from returning to homelessness, it is important not to lose sight of the problem of homelessness in the way that earlier medical-based explanations did. It is possible almost to be carried away by the descriptions of the prevalence of mental health problems, the high levels of alienation and the number of support needs in comparison with the general population and to start viewing single homeless people as unique. In fact, examining the characteristics of any relatively deprived section of society will yield comparable results to an examination of a group of single homeless people. Compare the health status of homeless people with that of council tenants in a deprived area and the similarities are strong, though one group is housed and the other is not (Victor 1992).

There is also a danger that *all* single homeless people are seen as individuals with a host of needs, which is clearly not the case; the prevalence of health problems and the extent of alienation may be high, but that is not the same thing as its being universal. Categorising single homeless people as vulnerable victims, which it is possible to do in many cases, also means that the individuals who are homeless are lost from sight. No one homeless person is quite like any other homeless person, and reducing individuals and their needs to categories does ultimately dehumanise them and mean that there is a danger of producing generalist policy responses based on a false understanding that ultimately suit no one. Homelessness cannot be reduced to relative health status, poverty, education or alienation, but it can be described as an *exclusion from society* that may require services ranging from the simple provision of adequate housing through to a package of housing, health, community care and social support services.

NOTES

1 See Pleace (1995) for further details. The research was funded by the Joseph Rowntree Foundation.

Chapter 12

Opening doors in the private rented sector
Developments in assistance with access

Julie Rugg

Ease of access is often regarded as a key characteristic of private renting, distinguishing the sector from the other tenures. Access to social housing is regulated by restrictive criteria which ensure that stock is allocated to households in greatest need. Although the government promotes owner occupation, the possibility of owning a home is only open to households with capital and a steady income. By contrast, renting privately is theoretically a tenure available to anyone able to pay the rent. Even households on low income can rent privately, since they are usually eligible for housing benefit that covers the cost of an average rent on a property appropriate to the size of the household. The government has repeatedly expressed its belief that private renting is a suitable tenure for single homeless people. However, for many single homeless people who are on benefits, securing a private rented letting is a process strewn with substantial obstacles: the supply of suitable accommodation is not always good; landlords are often unwilling to let to people on housing benefit; the benefit does not always cover the cost of the rent charged; it may be difficult to afford the rent in advance and deposit fees that many landlords require; and the often poor quality of property at the lower end of the market limits choice.

The last five years have seen the prolific development of a range of schemes that aim to help people overcome these difficulties. Accommodation registers help people find affordable accommodation of reasonable standard; deposit schemes help with the payment of bonds, either through cash loans or offering indemnities to landlords; and rent in advance schemes deal with the requirement to pay some rent up front. All these types of schemes are referred to in this chapter as 'access schemes', and can be defined in broad terms as schemes which help people secure independent private rented accommodation in tenancies intended to last at least six months. Government policy underlines the value of access schemes. Support for voluntary-sector agencies wanting to give this sort of help is available through the s.73 grant programme (Oldman, this volume). The programme – established under Section 73 of the 1985 Housing Act – gives grants to voluntary sector agencies that deliver services to non-statutorily homeless people. Grants are given for resettlement and outreach work, but the programme has increasingly prioritised funding for schemes giving access assistance. S.73 funds are not available to local authorities, but these have been encouraged to act by the issuing of a general consent that allows local authorities to set up funds to meet advance payments of rent or deposits.

Despite the consensus underlining the value of this sort of work, until recently very little was known about the way in which these schemes operate. In 1994 the Joseph Rowntree Foundation funded a detailed evaluation of access work. The research methods included a survey of 161 schemes operating in England and Wales, and interviews with project managers, clients and landlords. This chapter discusses findings from the research (reported fully in Rugg 1996). The first section describes the difficulties faced by people wanting to secure private rented accommodation. The second section discusses the characteristics of access schemes. The third section details the way in which schemes have responded to obstacles preventing people from renting privately. The final section discusses constraints which undermine the effective delivery of access assistance, and the conclusion offers some comments on the future of access work.

DIFFICULTIES WITH ACCESS TO PRIVATE RENTED ACCOMMODATION

A study of renting at the lower end of the market in Glasgow found that the majority of a sample of tenants, boarders and hostel residents (69 per cent) agreed with the statement that 'it is very difficult to find accommodation these days' (Kemp and Rhodes 1994). There are a number of problems facing people wanting to secure private rented accommodation. The problems overlap to some degree, but it is worth taking time to detail each in turn. This section of the chapter will, therefore, look at: the limited supply of appropriate accommodation; landlords' letting preferences; the affordability of private renting; the requirement to pay rent in advance and deposits; and the variable quality of property at the bottom end of the rental market.

In 1991 there was a major survey of single homeless people who were living in hostels and bed and breakfast (B&B) hotels, and who used day centres and soup runs. These people were asked about the problems which they had encountered in trying to find somewhere to rent. For many people, one of the principal obstacles was the lack of available accommodation. Over 80 per cent of those interviewed said that they wanted their own independent accommodation, where they did not have to share facilities. One hostel-user commented: 'I'm not asking for a palace, a small place with one bedroom, one kitchen, one bathroom, that I don't have to share with other people.' As the next chapter demonstrates, however, the flow of single-person, self-contained accommodation is limited compared with family-sized properties, which single people would not be able to afford to rent on their own. Thus accommodation suitable for single people is limited. This situation is exacerbated in some areas by competition for such property from other groups. For example, accommodation for single people may be especially poor in towns and cities with a high student population. An unpublished study of student accommodation in York found that many landlords preferred to let to students and were unlikely to let outside that niche market (Rugg et al. 1995).

Many people on low incomes are disadvantaged in any competition for property by the fact that many landlords are unwilling to let to people on housing benefit. In a survey of private landlords in Britain, Crook et al. (1995) found that most landlords judged prospective tenants by their economic status. Forty-nine per cent of landlords most preferred to let to people in work, and 29 per cent said that they least preferred to let to unemployed people. A survey of Scottish landlords found that seven in ten private individual landlords preferred tenants who were not in receipt of housing benefit (Kemp and Rhodes 1994). In explaining their preferences, some landlords mentioned the fact that they considered housing benefit claimants to be 'undesirable' in some way. For the majority, however, the decision not to take people on housing benefit rested with difficulties with the benefit system itself. In particular, mention was made of problems with applications and the lengthy time taken to process the benefit. Although local authorities are statutorily bound to process a claim within two weeks, delays do occur. For example, a study by Kemp and McLaverty (1995) found that almost half the private tenants in their survey had waited for between one and three months for their benefit to be paid. Landlords interviewed as part of the access scheme evaluation also expressed dissatisfaction with the housing benefit system. In particular, problems with overpayments of benefit were cited, and some landlords mentioned instances of having to pay back substantial amounts of benefit because tenants had not informed the benefits agency of changes in circumstances. It is these difficulties that lay behind the decision of many landlords to advertise properties with the stipulation 'no DSS'.

The attitude of landlords is one of the main difficulties attached to private renting, but the inaccessibility of private renting also has a financial aspect. The 1991 survey of single homeless people asked what problems they had encountered in trying to secure rented accommodation. The most frequently reported difficulty was that they felt that they simply could not afford to rent privately (Anderson *et al.* 1993). The 1993/94 Survey of English Housing showed that for most people with difficulties finding a place to stay, affordability was the main problem (Carey 1995). Research on the ability of the private rented sector (PRS) to house the homeless (upon which Chapter 13 is based) showed that rent levels in the PRS were consistently higher than social housing lettings. The mean rent per week of a private letting was £72, compared with a local authority letting at £39 and a housing association letting at £48 (Bevan and Rhodes 1996).

In principle, the level of the rent charged should not be a deterrent to people on low incomes wanting to rent, since it is possible for housing benefit to cover this cost entirely. However, the way in which the system operates means that there is often a shortfall between the rent charged and the benefit payable, and payment of this shortfall is the responsibility of the tenant. The shortfall may occur because the household is in accommodation that is too large for its needs, or the rent charged includes ineligible items such as heating or hot water. Shortfalls may also occur because the rent has been judged by the Rent Officer to be higher than the local average rent for comparable properties (the 'reference rent'). Housing benefit will not be paid in full on rents charged above the reference rent level. It is frequently the case that people in receipt of housing benefit can find themselves in tenancies where they are required to meet substantial shortfall payments. In 1994, a study of housing benefit claimants revealed that 40 per cent of claims were restricted, and average shortfall payments were up to £32 a week (Kemp *et al.* 1994). At present it is uncertain how the new reference rent has affected shortfall payments, since the regulation only came into force in January 1996. However, it is likely that average payments will have increased.

In addition to the possibility of housing benefit not covering the whole of the rent charged by the landlord, people on low income face other financial obstacles. Many landlords require tenants to pay some rent up front: the 1993/94 Survey of English Housing found that 73 per cent of tenants had made payments of rent in advance (Carey 1995). A 1990 survey of housing need in Cardiff found that over half the people interviewed said that they could not afford to pay rent in advance (Bailey 1992). Statutory help with rent in advance is available. People in receipt of Income Support can apply to the Social Fund for a grant or loan to cover rent in advance. Indeed, provision for this sort of payment was recommended by the Social Security Advisory Committee of 1992, which recognised in its report that people on Income Support 'frequently have no resources with which to pay large sums for rent in advance' (Social Security Advisory Committee 1992). However, there is evidence that few people approach the Social Fund for this purpose – possibly because for those who do, the success rate is limited. The Social Fund has a limited budget, and rent in advance payments are rarely prioritised. A report evaluating the Social Fund, published in 1992, found that less than 1 per cent of applications to the fund in its sample area were for rent in advance (Huby and Dix 1992). The survey of tenants at the lower end of the private sector in Glasgow revealed that only 7 per cent of people in its survey (who had moved since 1988) had applied to the Social Fund. Within this small group the success rate was low: two-thirds of applicants had been refused, and only one-quarter received assistance – usually through a loan (Kemp and Rhodes 1994). Help with rent in advance evidently has a low priority for many Social Fund administrators, but even in areas where assistance was relatively easy to secure, some problems remained. Interviews took place with access scheme clients in an area where payment of Social Fund loans for rent in advance was common. Claimants still felt constrained in their intentions to apply to the fund, since it was thought unlikely that payments would be made in cases when the rent was high. One access scheme client described her experience with the Social Fund:

> They'll ask for four weeks' rent in advance, and sometimes the rent might be £85 a week, or £95, and there's no way the social will give you that £400 because they'll say 'no it's too high'. So you can be left in limbo-land.

Thus, despite the theoretical availability of assistance, actual help can be difficult to secure.

In addition to rent in advance, landlords also often ask for deposits to cover any damage, theft or rent arrears accrued during the course of the tenancy. Sixty-three per cent of tenants in the Survey of English Housing had paid a deposit or non-returnable fee (Carey 1995). The requirement to pay a deposit is a considerable obstacle for people on low incomes. Over half the people in the 1990 survey of housing need in Cardiff said that the requirement to pay a deposit made it difficult to find accommodation (Bailey 1992). Qualitative interviews with access scheme clients found the same. Most of the clients said that bond payments were a big factor in their housing decisions, and in some cases was the biggest obstacle: 'that's what stops people from getting places to live'. Unlike rent in advance, there is no statutorily available assistance with bonds. Help had been available under the earlier single payments scheme but was removed in 1988, with the introduction of the Social Fund. The rationale behind this decision was the claim that both tenants and landlords had been abusing the scheme: expenditure on deposits had increased rapidly and by 1986–87 had reached £6.1m (Saunders 1991). Thus, despite the insuperable nature of this obstacle for many people, statutory assistance with deposits is not available. Local authorities are empowered to set up schemes to help with deposits and rent in advance, but the giving of assistance is not mandatory and the provision of assistance across the country remains patchy.

In their attempts to overcome financial obstacles, many people on low incomes look for accommodation at the bottom end of the market, where landlords are less likely to ask for advance payments. However, according to many of the access scheme clients, looking for somewhere to stay at the bottom end of the sector entailed an extensive search through any number of poor-quality properties. Exercising choice became an assessment of which property was the least bad. One access scheme client described her search:

> Some of the places me and my husband had been looking at were horrible and it was 'Eeeuuughhh'. You know, you wouldn't let pigs never mind humans live in there. So it has been a battle between finding places like that and some not wanting people on the Social or you had to be working.

For many people, securing renting accommodation became a trade-off: taking substandard property because the landlord did not ask for advance payments, and was willing to let to someone on benefits.

Thus for many people on low incomes there is little truth in the assumption that private renting can be characterised as a tenure of easy access. The supply of suitable accommodation is not always good; landlords operate restrictive criteria on people to whom they are willing to let; rents are not always affordable, even where housing benefit is available; advance payments are impossible to meet; and the quality of properties limits choice. The impact of this range of access difficulties on individual households is an intensification of housing need. People looking to rent privately do not always have the time to undertake a protracted search for suitable, reasonable quality, affordable accommodation where access is easy. Interviews with access scheme clients showed that many people who were looking for accommodation needed to find somewhere quickly: for example, one woman was escaping domestic violence; some clients were coming to the end of tenancies that the landlord was not renewing; one client had been living with a partner, and the relationship had broken down. For all these people, failure to secure somewhere to stay might mean having to persuade friends or relatives to let them stay temporarily, or in more extreme circumstances, having to move into a hostel or sleep on the street.

ACCESS SCHEMES

The establishment and growth of access schemes has been a remarkable development in the provision of services to people in housing need. The development has been a recent one: the majority of schemes have been set up since 1991. The spread of schemes has included two surges of activity. In 1991 more than double the number of schemes were set up compared with the previous year. This growth probably reflected the changes to s.73 funding, which for the first time made grants available to small voluntary-sector agencies wanting to set up individual projects to help homeless people in their area. The grants were targeted at schemes which set up accommodation registers. There was another doubling of schemes in 1993. This increase in numbers was largely due to a rapid rise in the popularity of deposit guarantee schemes, which in turn was perhaps a consequence of the increased availability of information on how to set up such schemes that was made available through the publication of the *Rent Guarantee Scheme Handbook* (Jenn 1993). During 1993 and 1994, the Joseph Rowntree evaluation attempted to draw together information on all schemes which were operating. It was evident that the speed of development was considerable. Contact information was collected for over 200 schemes, and 161 responded to a postal survey. Since April 1994, when the postal survey was completed, the number of schemes has continued to increase. Indeed, in 1995 a national forum representing deposit guarantee schemes was set up, and now has a full-time development worker. Although there is a consensus on the need for schemes, data from the postal survey showed that schemes were characterised by considerable diversity. This section of the chapter discusses their organisational arrangement, funding, types of client helped and dealings with the rental market.

The schemes were not uniform in terms of their parent organisation or the way in which they operated. Over half the schemes in the sample (56 per cent) were set up by voluntary-sector agencies. In many cases the scheme was being established as a complement to other services already being provided by the agency. Thus, for example, a hostel may secure funding for a worker to help residents to move into private rented accommodation. Another typical scenario was accommodation help being provided by an agency with a long-standing history of giving welfare advice: as more inquiries were received about difficulties with securing accommodation, so the agency made the decision to seek funding for a dedicated worker to run an accommodation register. There was a small number of schemes which were 'stand alone' and tended to work in collaboration with other agencies in their area. For example, the scheme might simply provide deposit assistance, but take referrals from agencies which themselves helped clients find somewhere to stay and offer support in settling in. Thirty per cent of schemes were run by local authorities. Here, two different ways of working were evident. In some instances, accommodation register projects were attached to housing advice offices. In other cases, the scheme might comprise help with advance payment which was given to non-priority statutory homeless households to help them move into private-sector accommodation.

The majority of the local authority schemes were funded from their housing department's general revenue budget. The funding picture was more complex for the voluntary-sector schemes, most which were dependent on a patchwork of funding from a range of different agencies. Nearly a third of voluntary-sector schemes had s.73 grants which covered 100 per cent of their revenue costs. It was more common for schemes to have only a proportion of their funding from the s.73 grant programme, since the funding is intended to last only three years and covers 90 per cent of revenue costs in the second year and 50 per cent in the third year. A typical voluntary-sector scheme, therefore, had a proportion of funding from s.73, and the remainder funded by charitable trusts, private donations or grants from the local authority. Most of the voluntary-sector schemes had annual incomes below £30,000, and those with money set aside to cover the issuing of guarantees had funds below £10,000.

Diversity was also evident in the scale at which schemes were operating. The survey requested information from each scheme on the number of clients it had helped in 1993/94. Some caution needed to be exercised in assessing returns since it was clear that definitions of 'helped' were not consistent. For some schemes, a client helped included all those to whom housing advice had been given. Other schemes only counted clients who had been given bonds or loans. Schemes offering financial help with deposits tended to help fewer clients, on average. This was perhaps because the work was often more formalised – for example, in the requirements to complete inventories – and the number of clients helped was limited by the cash available in the deposit fund. In particular, local authority deposit schemes helped the fewest clients, on average, with some schemes reporting that they had helped fewer than ten clients in the specified year. Many of these schemes reported that their assistance had been unpopular with the clients they were targeting – non-priority statutorily homeless households on the waiting list – who preferred to wait for a council tenancy. The largest numbers of clients helped were those assisted by voluntary-sector schemes offering quite informal advice in securing private rented accomodation. For example, the sample included some schemes which issued lists of vacancies compiled from local newspapers and from landlords contacting schemes with information. In these cases, the lists were freely available to anyone looking for accommodation, and so the spread of assistance was very wide.

As has been intimated, schemes differed in the types of client they were helping. Over 80 per cent of the schemes operated some sort of restriction in the type of client they assisted: for example, many only took local people on low incomes who were eligible for housing benefit. There was some degree of polarisation according to the type of organisation running the scheme. Voluntary-sector schemes were more likely to be helping single people, young people and people who were non-statutorily homeless. Local authority schemes were more likely to be restricting their help to families, people who were statutorily homeless, and people on the council waiting list. Taking both types of organisation together, a third only helped people who were capable of independent living. This restriction was often imposed because the schemes did not have a dedicated resettlement worker, did not think the PRS suitable for vulnerable clients, and did not deal with landlords who would be willing to take clients with, for example, disabilities or dependency problems.

As schemes differed in the sorts of client they helped, it was also clear that they did not all aim to secure accommodation in the same sector of the rental market. At least three distinct types of approach were evident. Some schemes were operating at the bottom end of the PRS, and dealt largely with landlords offering bedsits and rooms with shared kitchens and bathrooms, and were used to taking housing benefit clients. Landlords viewed the schemes as a good source of prospective tenants. Other schemes aimed for landlords towards the better-quality, self-contained sector of the market. These landlords were less likely to want to take housing benefit clients, but could be persuaded by the provision of rent in advance, bonds, assistance with housing benefit, and assurances that the scheme would 'keep an eye on' the client. Another type of relationship was also evident, between schemes and what has been termed 'reluctant landlords', who perhaps have only one property to let and are letting until the owner-occupied housing market revives. This type of landlord viewed the scheme as a proxy letting agent, in providing tenants, setting up the legal side of the tenancy and again dealing with the housing benefit.

Thus generalisation about access schemes on an organisational level is inadvisable. In addition to a basic distinction between schemes being run by local authorities and voluntary-sector agencies, there were also distinctions according to the type of client helped and the type of rental market in which the scheme aimed to operate.

ACCESS SCHEME SERVICES

Despite their diverse characteristics all access schemes helped their clients overcome the obstacles to private renting by using a range of strategies. This section of the chapter describes some of the ways in which the schemes aimed to sidestep individual difficulties.

The supply of rented accommodation

Most schemes attempted to increase the supply of rented accommodation to their clients. There were three sorts of approaches. Some schemes offered advice and services to 'reluctant landlords' and were actively advertising for properties which would have been new to the rental market, so increasing the overall net supply of rental accommodation. In addition there were examples of schemes which established relationships with builders, and were guaranteeing tenants for new developments, again increasing the amount of property on the market. It was more common, however, for schemes to try and increase the property available to their clients by contacting landlords who would not normally let to this client group. These landlords might be, for example, letting to students or only dealing in tourist trade.

Unwillingness of landlords to let to people on housing benefit

Many schemes spent time liaising with landlords and letting agents in their area, giving information on their particular scheme and trying to overcome landlord prejudices about benefit claimants. Some schemes countered prejudices by introducing landlords to prospective tenants, and offering to 'police' tenancies – keeping an eye on the property and dealing with clients if they caused any trouble. Schemes also provided services which removed difficulties that landlords might anticipate in letting to someone on benefit. Thus almost all schemes took responsibility for ensuring that the initial application was completed correctly, in order to minimise delays. Some schemes also set up a 'fast-tracking' system to ensure that payments would be paid within a given period of time; took responsibility for liaising with the housing benefit department on any queries; and dealt with any benefit appeals.

Affordability

Schemes saw that there was little point in setting up tenancies which then might fail because the client was unable to pay any shortfalls accruing from housing benefit payments being less than the contractual rent. In many cases, therefore, the scheme took over the task of compiling information on vacancies where the landlord would not insist on the shortfall payment being met, or were charging rents where a shortfall would not occur. Again this sort of work often included liaising with landlords and letting agents to give information on likely housing benefit payments, and making them more aware that clients would get into difficulties if large shortfall payments were insisted on. Schemes often stressed that they could provide a regular supply of tenants if the landlord charged a lower rent, thus minimising any losses the landlord might experience due to long-standing voids in properties.

Rent in advance

Some schemes dealt directly with the requirement to meet rent in advance payments, by offering a loan to cover the amount, which was then recovered from the first housing benefit cheque. Many more schemes, however, dealt with this payment less directly, by negotiating with the landlord to waive the requirement. In some cases the negotiation rested on scheme assurances that the landlord would receive the housing benefit payment more quickly by having a scheme tenant – because the application would be fast-tracked, for example.

Deposits

Assistance with deposit payments was more varied. In some cases the scheme paid the bond to the landlord on behalf of the client, and then required repayment once the tenancy ended. In other cases, the scheme paid the bond and then expected the tenant to reimburse the cost of the bond to the scheme by making small weekly payments. Other schemes sidestepped the requirement to hand over cash by offering to the landlord a written guarantee, which promised reimbursement for damage and theft, and in some cases also rent arrears and rent in lieu of notice. The guarantee was usually limited to a maximum payment – often the value of four weeks' rent. For many schemes, giving a guarantee meant that bond funds could be stretched, since bonds in excess of the value of the fund were issued on the expectation that only a certain percentage of claims would be made. Furthermore, the scheme did not then have the task of recovering cash payments from either tenant or landlord at the end of the tenancy – a difficulty which many cash deposit schemes acknowledged as the main failing of this way of working. Some schemes also negotiated with the landlord to reduce the amount of deposit required. This strategy did succeed, but often only with landlords at the lower-quality end of the market and offering shared accommodation, who again might want a quick turnover of clients to offset losses due to voids.

Poor-quality accommodation

Many schemes aimed to increase the choice of accommodation open to their clients by working to improve the quality of properties at the bottom end of the market. In some cases, the local authority schemes worked in conjunction with the local environmental health office, reporting landlords with substandard accommodation and only using shared accommodation which had been registered as fit by the local authority. Many schemes advised landlords on their statutory require- ments with respect to such aspects as gas and fire safety. Schemes often compiled vacancy lists which only included landlords whom they knew had good management practices, such as responding quickly to requests for repairs. Landlords offering substandard properties were excluded. Schemes also encouraged landlords in the better-quality, self-contained market to let to scheme clients by using a range of financial inducements, including payment of bonds and rent in advance, and dealing with housing benefit.

Thus schemes operated specific strategies which countered the obstacles facing people who wanted to rent privately. It should be stressed that schemes rarely offered a single service. More often, they offered groups of services which together ensured that someone was given access to vacant properties, that help was offered with advance payments, and that follow-up support was available, at least in the few weeks following the start of the tenancy. Thus scheme response to the difficulties of access was largely holistic. Furthermore, most schemes tailored the services they offered to accommodate the characteristics of the rental market in their area, and the type of clients they were helping.

In addition, it should be noted that the majority of schemes also went beyond the provision of an immediate response to these obsta- cles, and also offered services that aimed to enhance a tenancy's sustainability. Much of this side of access work connects with a tenancy's affordability, but other things are also considered. Many schemes, for example, ensured that tenancies were established with a legally binding tenancy agreement, which established the right of the tenant to stay in the property for a specified period. For many schemes, however, the main task of ensuring a tenancy's sustain- ability lay in continued services once a tenancy had been set up. For example, visits to clients took place following the start of the ten- ancy to ensure that the tenant had settled in, and to advise on bud- geting to pay gas, electricity and other bills. The schemes also liaised between the tenant and the landlord on such issues as repairs. The schemes thus retained a mediating role to ensure that situations did not arise which could lead to a breakdown in the tenancy.

This section has shown that access schemes used a range of strategies to counter access obstacles, and in doing so intended to provide a 'seamless' service that covered all potential problems simultaneously. Access work also had a preventive aspect, in aiming to set up tenancies which were sustainable, thus providing a long-term solution to housing need. Despite the positive contribution schemes can make to the alleviation of non-statutory single homelessness in particular, there are factors which operate to limit their effectiveness. The final section of the chapter discusses some of these constraints.

CONSTRAINTS ON ACCESS WORK

The postal survey asked schemes about the difficulties they had with their work, and five key problems were highlighted. Many schemes commented that, despite a range of strategies, there was still an unwillingness amongst landlords to let to scheme clients. This was reported as a problem by 55 per cent of schemes. In many cases, schemes were able to liaise successfully with landlords in their area, but the offer of scheme services was not always sufficient inducement. For example, some landlords were unwilling to respond because they already had an established tenant base and the supply of tenants was good. Many schemes said that their clients had little hope of securing a tenancy when there were people in the market for similar properties who were employed, and who could pay cash up front and regular rent without having to wait for the housing benefit to be processed.

An associated problem was difficulties with delays in housing benefit payments, which was frequently or constantly a problem for 45 per cent of schemes. Although some schemes were able to set up fast-tracking systems, and have their claims prioritised by the local benefits agency, not all schemes could work in this way. In some instances, schemes were working with housing benefit offices which were deemed to be particularly inefficient. Even where schemes were careful to submit correctly completed application forms, delays in payment could sometimes last weeks. Since most schemes used a 'speeded-up' housing benefit payment as their main inducement to landlords to take scheme clients as tenants, scheme effectiveness could be limited in areas where the housing benefit office would not co-operate.

A further problem, experienced constantly or frequently by 40 per cent of schemes, was the support needs of the clients with whom they dealt. For many schemes, support might simply include ensuring that the client had settled in during the first few weeks of the tenancy. In other cases, however, the support need was more intensive. Some schemes recognised the difficult choices to be made with respect to taking on the more problematic clients. Taking on such people without resettlement support would probably lead to failed tenancies and landlords who might refuse to take any further scheme clients as tenants. However, not taking on such people would lead to that group's becoming further marginalised. Consequently, securing funding for resettlement workers has become a priority for many schemes.

A fourth problem, experienced by 62 per cent of schemes, was the need to secure long-term funding. This problem was particularly acute amongst voluntary-sector schemes, 83 per cent of which said that securing funding was constantly or frequently a problem. At the heart of this difficulty was the fact that many of these schemes were established on time-limited s.73 funding. The intention of the funding programme was to 'kick-start' schemes in areas where need was evident. The funding was given on the expectation that after three years the schemes would have proved their worth and so be able to secure grants from the local authority, businesses, or from charitable trusts. As one manager commented, however, 'the government seems to think this is going to happen. I see no evidence of it'. Indeed, many schemes found it difficult to secure support after the initial enthusiasm of setting up a new scheme had settled. According to one project worker:

> Some of the big charities like CRISIS, Children in Need, said initially they didn't mind starting you off – starting off a new project. But now they're looking to fund other new projects and what they're saying is, 'Well, if you're so vital to the local scene, the local authority should be funding you.' But unfortunately the local authority might think, yes we're very vital, but they haven't got any money because they're hitting budgets and having cuts and so there's no funding from them either.

Follow-up interviews with project managers during the summer of 1996 showed that many had gone back for s.73 funding for 'another' worker, with a repackaged job description. Some schemes had secured funding from the National Lottery, but in general, levels of insecurity remained high. Although the value of access work has been widely recognised, appreciation has not grown to the extent that long-term funding for such work is easily available.

The biggest constraint, which was reported as being constantly or frequently a problem for 79 per cent of schemes, was the limited availability of affordable, reasonable quality accommodation. Many project managers reported bottlenecks of clients who had been assessed but for whom no place to stay was available. The success of access work is heavily reliant on a good supply of accommodation, which in itself depends on the characteristics of the local rental market. As the next chapter demonstrates, rental markets differ in their ability to respond to extra demand. In some cases there may never have been a particularly strong tradition of private renting, or the physical characteristics of the rental market prove to be problematic. For example, in some areas accommodation available for rent is largely in the form of two-bedroomed terraced houses, unsuitable for letting as single accommodation. It may also be the case that the little accommodation that is available is of poor condition. Many schemes will not place people in property where the state of repair is unsatisfactory, since it is unlikely that tenants will want to stay there for any length of time. Follow-up interviews with scheme managers in August 1996 showed that for the vast majority, limited accommodation was still their biggest problem, even after a year of actively promoting an increased supply of property.

CONCLUSION: THE FUTURE OF ACCESS WORK

This chapter has shown that considerable difficulties face people trying to secure access to private rented accommodation. The last five years have seen the development of a range of schemes that are able to respond in a flexible way to these problems, and to operate in a preventive role by aiming to set up sustainable tenancies which provide a long-term solution to an individual's housing need. The chapter has shown that at the time at which the fieldwork was completed, there were some constraints evident on schemes' ability to respond to client's needs: landlords' unwillingness to let to scheme clients and limitations in the supply of accommodation were both particularly problematic. Since that time, however, there have been changes which indicate that the access work may be further constrained. One anticipated effect of the 1996 Housing Act will be increased demand for private sector accommodation (Bevan and Rhodes, this volume). It has been shown that scheme tenants do not always fare well when there is competition for property from other sources.

The position of scheme tenants is exacerbated by the fact that many of them are under the age of twenty-five. From October 1996, housing benefit for the majority of under-twenty-fives was restricted to the value of shared accommodation. Interviews with scheme managers in the summer of 1996 found that some landlords, uncertain how the changes will affect the rents they charge, were already showing an increased unwillingness to let to this client group. Schemes that have in the past sought to find self-contained dwellings for their young clients are now actively encouraging landlords to let their property as shared accommodation. It can only be concluded that help with access, the basic structure of which has only recently been developed, is already facing the need for major revision.

Chapter 13

The capacity of the private rented sector to house homeless households

Mark Bevan and David Rhodes

The aim of the research reported here was to provide an evaluation of the capacity and appropriateness of the private rented sector (PRS) to house statutorily homeless people.[1] The original motivation for the research was the Green Paper *Access to Local Authority and Housing Association Tenancies: A Consultation Paper* (DoE 1994a), outlining the government's intentions for changes to the homelessness legislation, and the subsequent responses to the proposals. It was felt by the researchers that an independent evaluation of the existing evidence could help inform the policy debate, which at that time was highly politicised. Since the completion of the research, of course, there has been the subsequent housing White Paper (DoE 1995a), and the resulting Housing Act 1996 received Royal Assent on 24 July 1996 (Lowe, this volume).

The research was comprised of two parts. The first of these was an evaluation of the appropriateness of the PRS to house statutorily homeless people, which involved an examination of existing relevant research and statistics. The second part of the research comprised an analysis of the capacity of the PRS to house the homeless, which took as its starting point the 1991 Census.[2] This chapter contains a discussion of the second part of the research. Many of the issues relevant to the evaluation of the appropriateness of the PRS to house the homeless are discussed in Rugg (this volume) and Bevan and Rhodes (1997).

BACKGROUND TO THE RESEARCH

Statutory homelessness was defined under Part III of the Housing Act 1985, and remains broadly the same under the new legislation (Lowe, this volume). A household is statutorily homeless if it satisfies four criteria: it is homeless or threatened with homelessness within twenty-eight days; there is a priority need; the household must not be intentionally homeless; and there is a local connection.

Prior to the Housing Act 1996, local authorities were required to provide the households they accepted as statutorily homeless with secure tenancies, usually in housing association or council housing accommodation. Homeless acceptances were usually given priority for housing, research showing that on average they were housed about twice as quickly as other applicants (Prescott-Clarke *et al.* 1994). Homeless households generally had, however, less choice of accommodation, frequently being given just one offer of housing, whereas non-homeless applicants on housing waiting lists were often given the option of refusing up to two reasonable offers before incurring a penalty (Bines *et al.* 1993).

The Green Paper proposed changes to the way in which social rented housing should be allocated. The main thrust of the proposals have remained intact in the 1996 Act, and were based on the premise that the existing method of allocating social rented housing was on an unfair basis:

> Ministers see no good reason why a person accepted as statutorily homeless should have priority in the allocation of what is in effect housing for life over people who remain in unsatisfactory accommodation until their turns come up on a waiting list.
>
> (DoE 1994a: Para 2.8)

Thus the 'fast-track' priority given to the homeless has been removed, with local authorities being required to operate a single general waiting list for all applicants. Local authorities have to provide temporary accommodation for the homeless to tide them over their immediate crisis, and which the government believes will allow them sufficient time to secure their own longer-term housing. The 1996 Act has extended the requirement for temporary provision for a period of up to two years, from the initially proposed six months. A key element of the provision of temporary housing for the homeless is the government's emphasis on increased use of the PRS to perform this function, thus raising the question of whether the PRS has the capacity to take on this role.

The Green Paper received an unprecedented number of responses, most of which were in opposition to the proposed changes. Aside from the view that there was no evidence of a need for change, there were two broad themes to many of the responses. First, there were arguments that the PRS was not an appropriate form of tenure for the homeless; and second, there were concerns that the sector did not have the capacity to take on the role of housing the homeless. It was these two themes that the research aimed to evaluate through an analysis of existing data and literature. The remainder of the chapter concentrates on the evaluation of the capacity of the PRS to house the homeless.

METHODS

The evaluation of the capacity of the PRS to house the statutorily homeless was based on an analysis of the 1991 Census. For the year 1994, it was possible to make a comparison of the number of statutorily homeless acceptances with the flows of PRS lettings and social rented lettings. The comparisons were made for all districts of England. The method employed in making the comparisons involved several stages, which are outlined below.

First, it was necessary to adjust the Census to account for the growth in the size of the PRS between April 1991 (when the Census was held) and December 1994. The *Housing and Construction Statistics* provide regional figures, the lowest level of disaggregation available, on the stock of private rented dwellings. From these figures the numbers of households in all districts of each respective region in the furnished and unfurnished PRS were estimated for 1994. For the whole of England, this procedure gave an estimated increase in the number of PRS households in the furnished and unfurnished subsectors from 1,396,768 at the time of the Census to 1,492,500 by the end of 1994 (equivalent to an average increase of approximately 7 per cent for England).

Second, to calculate the numbers of lettings likely to become available during 1994, it was necessary to estimate the flow of PRS lettings in the furnished and unfurnished subsectors. The turnover of lettings in the PRS was higher in the furnished than the unfurnished subsector: the *Survey of English Housing* (DoE 1995c) showed that the proportion of households remaining at the same PRS address for less than one year for the whole of England was 61 per cent for the furnished subsector, and 29 per cent for the unfurnished subsector. Analysis of the *Survey of English Housing* data files, however, provided figures for the furnished and unfurnished subsectors at a greater level of disaggregation, and which were used to estimate the flow of PRS lettings in each district for 1994.

Third, the evaluation was based on accommodation which was fit for human habitation, by making an allowance for levels of unfitness in the PRS. Regional figures for the level of unfitness were taken from the *English House Condition Survey* (DoE 1993), and applied to all districts in each respective region.

In total, it was estimated that in 1994 there was a total flow of 533,952 lets in the furnished and unfurnished PRS (and hence available to the public) which were within the fitness standard (Table 13.1). This figure comprised 36 per cent of the estimated total number of households renting privately in furnished and unfurnished accommodation in 1994. Greater London and the South East had the largest flows of lettings. The lowest estimated flow of lettings was in the North, a feature which was partly a function of the high level of unfitness in the region (31 per cent of the PRS in the North was classed as unfit, compared with an average of 21 per cent for England as a whole).

It has been suggested that a number of tenancies in the unfurnished PRS for formerly homeless people have broken down because of their need for furniture (Jenn 1994). Equally, many statutorily homeless households will have their own furniture and will require unfurnished dwellings, rather than having to sell or store their possessions. Thus, the needs of households will vary, making it important that the appropriate type of accommodation is available.

Table 13.2 shows that on average just over two-thirds of the flow of PRS lettings was in the furnished subsector and the remainder was in the unfurnished subsector. Three-quarters of the estimated flow of

Table 13.1 Estimated annual flow of PRS lettings in 1994 by region

| | Flow of PRS lettings | |
Region	*(No.)*	*(%)*
North	23,592	4
Yorkshire & Humberside	52,769	10
North West	54,734	10
West Midlands	38,894	7
East Midlands	39,253	7
East Anglia	25,184	5
South West	60,979	11
South East (excl. London)	101,625	19
Greater London	136,922	26
England	533,952	100

Source: 1991 Census. Own analysis

Table 13.2 Estimated annual flow of furnished and unfurnished lettings
by region

Region	Furnished (%)	Unfurnished (%)	Total (%)
North	64	36	100
Yorkshire & Humberside	66	34	100
North West	69	31	100
West Midlands	64	36	100
East Midlands	63	37	100
East Anglia	64	36	100
South West	68	32	100
South East (excl. London)	65	35	100
Greater London	75	25	100
England	68	32	100

Source: 1991 Census. Own analysis

lettings in Greater London were furnished. The proportion of furnished lettings across the other regions of England ranged between 63 per cent and 69 per cent. Rural areas on average had higher flows of unfurnished lettings than non-London urban areas (48 per cent and 31 per cent respectively).

THE AVAILABILITY OF LETTINGS FOR FAMILIES

Property size is an important consideration in the assessment of how appropriate the PRS may be to accommodate the homeless. Research on the Private Sector Leasing scheme (London Research Centre 1991) found that some local authorities had experienced difficulties in securing sufficient numbers of appropriately sized properties within their areas. Clearly, it would be inappropriate to accommodate households in lettings which were too small for their needs, such as families with children in one-bedroom properties. On the other hand, the concern was raised in the research on Private Sector Leasing that families which had been placed in over-large PRS accommodation, because of a shortage of smaller property, may be difficult to place subsequently in more appropriately sized permanent accommodation because of their changed expectations. Therefore, households' requirements in terms of property size need to be taken into account. Furthermore, over-accommodating households in receipt of housing benefit may result in a shortfall between their rent and the amount of assistance they receive.

The great majority of statutorily homeless acceptances are likely to be households comprising one or more adults with children (Prescott-Clarke *et al.* 1994). Therefore, property which has two or more bedrooms will be suitable for the majority of acceptances. The analysis considers PRS accommodation in terms of its size. As the Census contains counts of the number of rooms occupied, rather than a separate count of the number of bedrooms, dwellings suitable for housing families were defined in the research as comprising three or more rooms, one room being a living room and the two others bedrooms. However, some statutorily homeless households will be composed of single people or couples. Dwellings with one or two rooms were classed as suitable for single people or couples – that is, as comprising one bedroom. It was estimated that in total there was a flow of 410,306 dwellings in England that were available with two or more bedrooms, and hence suitable for accommodating families (accounting for 77 per cent of the estimated total flow of fit dwellings).

In all regions of the country there was a much higher estimated proportion of family-sized accommodation compared with accommodation with one bedroom. Table 13.1 above shows that the Greater London region had the largest flow of private lets (just over one-quarter of all lets in England). Table 13.3, however, shows that a lower proportion of these lets in the capital would have been large enough to house families compared with other regions. In particular, the proportion of private lets large enough for families in authorities

Table 13.3 Estimated regional flow of PRS lettings by number of bedrooms

Region	One bedroom (%)	Two or more bedrooms (%)	Total (%)
North	16	84	100
Yorkshire & Humberside	23	77	100
North West	25	75	100
West Midlands	20	80	100
East Midlands	18	82	100
East Anglia	17	83	100
South West	25	75	100
South East (excl. London)	21	79	100
Greater London	28	72	100
England	23	77	100

Source: 1991 Census. Own analysis

such as Islington and Camden was as low as 60 per cent. Table 13.3 suggests that it would have been easier to find family-sized accommodation in the North, the Midlands and East Anglia. Over four-fifths of private lets in these regions were large enough to accommodate family households. This proportion was even higher in a number of individual authorities. For example, 95 per cent of private lets in Castle Morpeth, in the county of Northumberland, were suitable for families.

On average, a larger proportion of furnished lettings were suitable for single people or couples compared with unfurnished lettings: three in ten furnished lettings were appropriately sized for single people and couples, whereas about one in ten unfurnished lettings was comprised of one bedroom.

THE CAPACITY OF THE PRS TO HOUSE HOMELESS HOUSEHOLDS

In order to illustrate the capacity of the PRS to cater for the demands which could be placed upon it by accommodating homeless households, this part of the chapter considers the relationship between the flow of private lettings in 1994 and the numbers of households accepted as statutorily homeless in the same year. Thus a local authority with a low estimated flow of PRS lettings may also have had a comparatively low number of homeless acceptances, and hence a relatively favourable capacity to house the homeless. The analysis was performed at the local authority level for all districts of England.

The analysis in this part of the chapter is based on the number of homeless acceptances as a proportion of the total flow of PRS lettings: the figures show the percentage of the estimated flow of lettings in the PRS which would have been used had all statutorily homeless acceptances been housed in the sector. Thus, a low percentage indicates that the PRS had a relatively large capacity compared with the number of homeless acceptances. Conversely, a high percentage indicates a low capacity of private lets in relation to the number of homeless acceptances. The calculation is intended to provide an indication of the capacity of the PRS to accommodate homeless households, as in practice only a proportion of homeless households are likely to be housed in the PRS.

On average, 23 per cent of the flow of lettings in the PRS in England would have been used if all homeless households were housed in the

Table 13.4 Estimated capacity of the PRS to house the homeless by
           region

Region	Mean (%)
North	29
Yorkshire & Humberside	20
North West	33
West Midlands	42
East Midlands	22
East Anglia	13
South West	15
South East (excl. London)	18
Greater London	21
England	23

Source: 1991 Census and DoE *(1995d) Information Bulletin*, London: HMSO.
Own analysis

sector in 1994. Table 13.4 shows that there were broad regional differences, with East Anglia and the South West having the largest
capacities to accommodate the statutorily homeless (13 per cent and
15 per cent of the flow of lettings would have been used), and the
West Midlands and the North West the lowest capacities (42 per cent
and 33 per cent of the flow of lettings would have been used).

The regional figures on the capacity of the PRS to house the homeless disguise a large amount of variation at the district level. The
proportion of private lets that would be used if all the homeless
were housed in the sector ranged from a low of 3 per cent in Fylde,
Blackpool and Torridge to a high of 198 per cent in Walsall. In other
words, there were about double the number of homeless acceptances
in Walsall as there were available lettings. There were a small number of other districts where the number of homeless acceptances in
1994 was much larger than the estimated total flow of privately
rented accommodation, including Tamworth, Halton and Redditch.
Local authorities tended to have a lower PRS capacity, particularly in
the North West and the West Midlands. These trends are reflected in
Table 13.5, which shows the districts with the highest and lowest
proportion of private lettings compared with homelessness acceptances. It is in local authorities where the PRS is small in relation to
levels of homelessness that local authorities' ability to utilise this
tenure to make inroads into accommodating the statutorily homeless
are likely to be most constrained.

Table 13.5 Local authorities with the highest and lowest estimated
PRS capacities to house the homeless

Local authority	Flow of PRS lettings (no.)	Homeless acceptances (no.)	Proportion of PRS which would be used (%)
Highest capacity			
Fylde	1,140	29	3
Blackpool	3,282	95	3
Torridge	838	29	3
Forest Heath	824	33	4
Southend on Sea	2,198	88	4
Great Yarmouth	1,293	56	4
Kettering	738	33	4
Alnwick	375	17	5
Exeter	1,896	88	5
Thanet	1,912	90	5
Lowest capacity			
Harlow	264	192	73
Tameside	1,165	912	78
Sedgefield	240	195	81
Chorley	388	358	92
Sandwell	1,242	1,225	99
Basildon	499	496	99
Redditch	347	361	104
Halton	421	439	104
Tamworth	250	268	107
Walsall	1,090	2,156	198

Sources: 1991 Census and DoE (1995d) *Information Bulletin*, London: HMSO.
Own analysis

HOMELESSNESS AND ACCESS TO ALL RENTED ACCOMMODATION

The Department of the Environment suggested that local authorities will be able to use a range of accommodation to meet the new duty to secure accommodation for a minimum of twelve months (now increased to two years) for a person accepted as unintentionally homeless: 'This may include accommodation within an authority's own stock (on a non-secure basis), accommodation in housing association stock (on an assured shorthold tenancy), placement with a private landlord, or a place in a special needs scheme' (DoE 1995a).

This part of the chapter considers the availability of tenancies in the PRS alongside the flow of lets in both local authority and housing association accommodation. The combination of the three types of rented accommodation gives an indication of the total opportunity for rehousing within individual local authorities. In particular, the analysis serves to indicate areas where the PRS could be used as an additional resource in instances where the flow of lettings in the social housing sector may be relatively low. The supply of re-lets in the local authority sector in 1993/94 was assessed using HIP1 returns[3] net of transfers and exchanges. These were added to the number of re-lets made by housing associations in each local authority area in 1993/94 (using HAR/10).[4]

In the final quarter of 1993/94, 42 per cent of housing association dwellings were single bedrooms or bedsits, and the Housing Corporation (1995) has suggested that the nature of the stock has constrained the ability of associations to alleviate statutory homelessness. Throughout 1993/94, however, one-third of housing association lettings were to homeless households. Two-thirds of these lettings were to statutorily homeless households under the terms of the 1985 Housing Act, whilst the remainder of them were to what the housing associations considered to be homeless households, although they did not meet the provisions of the 1985 Housing Act (Housing Corporation 1995).

The capacity of the social housing sector was expressed as the percentage of re-lets in 1993/94 which would have been absorbed if all homeless acceptances for 1994 had been housed in the sector. This calculation showed that, overall, 36 per cent of re-lets in the social housing sector would have been absorbed if all households accepted as statutorily homeless had been housed in this sector (Table 13.6). However, this proportion varied regionally, and just over two-fifths of re-lets in the social housing sector in Greater London would have been absorbed if all homeless acceptances had been housed in the sector. A similar situation was apparent in the West Midlands. In contrast, a much lower proportion of social housing re-lets would have been used in the North and East Anglia.

Table 13.6 also shows the impact of adding the estimated number of private lets to the total number of social lets upon the potential opportunity for rehousing statutorily homeless households. This procedure shows that, overall, the proportion of the total flow of lets which would have been used more than halved, from 36 per cent of the flow of social lettings to 13 per cent of all lettings. Furthermore, the addition of private lets to all social lets had a smoothing effect upon the level of variation between regions in terms of the proportion of all lets which would have been taken

Table 13.6 Homeless acceptances in 1994 as a proportion of social and PRS lettings

Region	Local authority & housing association lettings (%)	Local authority, housing association & PRS lettings (%)
North	21	12
Yorkshire & Humberside	27	12
North West	33	17
West Midlands	38	20
East Midlands	29	13
East Anglia	25	9
South West	40	11
South East (excl. London)	32	12
Greater London	41	14
England	36	13

Sources: 1991 Census, DoE Housing Investment Programme returns (HIP1 1993/94), DoE Housing Association Return, form 10 (HAR/10) and DoE (1995d) Information Bulletin, London: HMSO. Own analysis

by homeless households. Considering social lets only, the proportion which would have been used to house all homeless households varied by a range of 20 per cent across the regions (21 per cent in the North to 41 per cent in Greater London). With the addition of private lets, the range reduced to 11 per cent (the lowest being East Anglia with 9 per cent, and the West Midlands being the highest, with 20 per cent).

Table 13.6 also indicates those regions where the use of private lets would have the largest impact upon the opportunity for rehousing homeless households. On average, the PRS could make large contributions in Greater London and the South West. In Greater London, the proportion of lets which would have been absorbed by housing all homeless acceptances reduced from 41 per cent of all social lettings to 14 per cent of the combined total of social and PRS lettings. In the South West, the respective proportions were 40 per cent and 11 per cent. The region where the addition of PRS lets had the least impact upon the rehousing opportunities of local authorities was the North.

Table 13.7 lists local authorities with the highest and lowest estimated total rented capacities (PRS plus all social rented lettings) to house the homeless. The table shows that many districts are in similar rank order to those in Table 13.5 above, which lists districts in

Table 13.7 Local authorities with the highest and lowest total rented capacities to house the homeless

Local authority	Social & PRS lettings (no.)	Homeless acceptances 1994 (no.)	Proportion of the total flow of lettings used (%)
Highest capacity			
Fylde	1,309	29	2
Blackpool	4,030	95	2
Alnwick	630	17	3
Kettering	1,212	33	3
Southend on Sea	3,170	88	3
Torridge	1,000	29	3
Forest Heath	1,128	33	3
Great Yarmouth	1,760	56	3
Chiltern	1,521	49	3
Thanet	2,738	90	3
Lowest capacity			
Tameside	3,009	912	30
Bolton	3,554	1,082	30
Chorley	1,175	358	30
Tamworth	871	268	31
Bury	2,166	667	31
North-west Leicestershire	960	298	31
Basildon	1,538	496	32
Redditch	1,004	361	36
Broxbourne	793	303	38
Walsall	3,345	2,156	64

Sources: 1991 Census, HIP1 1993/94, HAR/10 1993/94 and DoE (1995d) *Information Bulletin*, London: HMSO. Own analysis

terms of the capacity of the PRS alone. Blackpool and Fylde had the most favourable total rented and PRS capacities to house the homeless, and Walsall stands out as having the smallest total rented and PRS capacities to house the homeless.

CONCLUSIONS

Table 13.4 has shown that authorities with the greatest private rented capacity relative to levels of statutory homelessness were in East Anglia, the South West and the South East. Local authorities would be most likely to have the greatest opportunity to make use of the PRS in these regions. Districts in the North West and the North, however, would be likely to have less scope for utilising the PRS in these regions, as the number of homeless acceptances was relatively high compared with the flow of private sector lettings.

Given the average size of the social rented sector compared with levels of statutory homelessness in Greater London, Table 13.6 suggests that the PRS could potentially make a large positive change to the overall capacity of local authorities in this area to house the homeless. This finding perhaps reflects the extent to which some London boroughs have already been using the PRS to accommodate homeless households temporarily (LRC 1991). In contrast, the PRS would be likely to have less of a positive impact in the North.

The regional variations presented in the chapter are averages for the local authorities in each region, and as such disguise a large amount of variation in the capacities at the district level. In addition, the estimations of capacity belie the extent to which a considerable proportion of the flow of lettings are unlikely to become available for homeless households for a range of reasons (Rugg, this volume), including the letting preferences of private landlords, the difficulty which tenants may experience in paying the higher rents in the PRS compared with the social rented sector, potential problems with affording payments of rent in advance and deposits, competition from groups of tenants who traditionally look to the PRS as a source of accommodation, and the existence of private landlords supplying niche markets and who are unlikely to consider diversifying.

In practice, local authorities have had mixed experiences of trying to encourage private landlords to house homeless households. Evans (1991) found that few local authorities reported difficulty in finding accommodation in the PRS when developing private sector leasing schemes to accommodate homeless households on a temporary basis. On the other hand, Rugg (1996) found that about two-thirds of local authorities operating access schemes for the PRS reported that they frequently or constantly experienced difficulties in finding adequate supplies of affordable accommodation of reasonable quality. In addition, Evans also found that some authorities have chosen not to rely too heavily on the PRS in case changes in market conditions lead to a fall in the level of lettings available, or if a large quantity of tenancies come to an end at the same time, thus placing an undue strain on the social housing sector.

The estimates of the capacity of the PRS, and the PRS plus social rented lettings, to house the homeless therefore only provide an indication of the likely housing opportunities for local authorities. The figures can do no more than provide estimates of the housing possibilities for homeless households in each district of England.

NOTES

1 The research was funded by the Joseph Rowntree Foundation. The authors gratefully acknowledge the guidance of Peter Kemp, who was the director of the research.
2 Material from Crown copyright records made available through the Office of Population Censuses and the ESRC Data Archive, has been used by permission of the controller of HM Stationery Office.
3 The annual Housing Investment Programme return by local authorities to the Department of the Environment covering basic housing management information.
4 The annual Housing Association Return made by housing associations to the Housing Corporation which covers basic housing management information.

Chapter 14

Hostels
A useful policy and practice response?

Joanne Neale

For many years, hostels have provided an important source of low-cost accommodation, frequently targeted at specific groups of people. These have included homeless families, single homeless people, ex-offenders, people with a learning difficulty and mothers and babies (Thomas and Niner 1989). It is, however, widely believed that hostels are a second-rate, inferior form of accommodation and that hostel residents are society's failures. Likewise, hostels tend to be associated with poor-quality buildings, insanitary conditions and institutionalised living arrangements, such as dormitory sleeping and communal dining. Compounding such negative associations, contemporary debates in community care frequently espouse 'independent living' and 'a home of one's own', rather than shared hostel living, as the preferred goal for all individuals.

If such values and assumptions are accepted without question, it seems unlikely that hostels will ever provide 'real homes' for their residents. Similarly, it suggests that hostels can only be of limited use as a policy and practice response to the problem of homelessness. The aim of this chapter is to question received wisdoms of this kind. To this end, the first part provides a brief history of hostel provision and the second presents some of the main findings from previous research on hostels and hostel residents. The third part then focuses on a recent qualitative study, conducted by the present author. This research allowed individuals with direct experience of hostel accommodation to speak for themselves and to describe hostel life in their own words. In so doing, it provided some useful insights into a range of topics which had hitherto received little attention.

The conclusion drawn from all three sections is that hostels are a very valuable policy and practical service response to homelessness. Consequently, there is a need to challenge negative stereotypes and to reappraise hostel accommodation more positively. This will, however, require evaluating both the qualitative and experiential aspects of hostel living (such as how it feels and what it means to live in a hostel), as well as the more quantitative and tangible features of provision (such as funding, standards, support services and staffing).

A HISTORY OF HOSTEL PROVISION

Before 1948, statutory provision for homeless people comprised the casual wards and workhouses, run by the Poor Law authorities and commonly known as 'spikes'. These were primitive and punitive forms of shelter which espoused the principles of less eligibility and individual blameworthiness. Only meagre assistance for the destitute was provided, and those who were not recognised as citizens of a particular parish could be evicted under the Vagrancy Acts and the laws of settlement (Donnison and Ungerson 1982; Watson and Austerberry 1986; Clapham *et al.* 1990). The non-statutory accommodation available to homeless people at that time was similarly very basic. It included Salvation Army hostels, Rowton houses, night shelters, common lodging houses and commercial hostels. This non-statutory provision was usually provided inside large converted warehouses, also on a direct access basis.

In 1948, the National Assistance Act abolished the Poor Law and most of the remaining casual wards were closed. A number were, however, maintained as short-stay 'reception centres' to be managed by the National Assistance Board (Watson and Austerberry 1986; Clapham *et al.* 1990). The ethos of the reception centres tended to be less punitive than that of the casual wards, but provision still emphasised the deviant characteristics of homeless people, rather than issues such as housing shortage (Watson and Austerberry 1986). Homeless people were, in the main, considered responsible for their situation and, consequently, deemed blameworthy and deserving of little more than basic standards and amenities, coupled with support and supervision (Evans 1991).

For many years, large, poor-quality, substandard hostels were the most common form of temporary accommodation used by local authorities. Provision was not considered worthy of any great financial investment from housing departments. In any case, there was frequently no money available to refurbish existing buildings or to develop alternatives (Watchman and Robson 1989; Evans 1991). The 1974 Housing Act, however, marked the beginning of an era of radical change in the hostel world. This Act made funding available to housing associations, via the Housing Corporation, to build new, or to modernise old, buildings on a large scale. Housing associations were seen as providing a 'useful supplementary resource' to local authority housing departments, and were particularly associated with the provision of 'special needs' accommodation. Consequently, many smaller, more specialised housing projects emerged (Canter *et al.* 1990; Watson and Cooper 1992). As a result, the stereotypical image of a hostel as a large, depersonalised building essentially offering only dormitory sleeping arrangements to older men with drink problems became increasingly irrelevant.

In addition to the 1974 Housing Act, other policies and initiatives subsequently pursued by central and local government brought further changes to the range of available hostel accommodation. The first of these was the 'Hostels Initiative', launched in 1980 by John Stanley, the then Housing Minister. Its objective was to improve the standard of temporary accommodation available to single homeless people by modernising or closing down the very large, traditional hostels and night shelters and replacing them with a more diverse range of smaller, higher-quality hostel provision (Anderson *et al.* 1993). Complementing this, a further important change to hostel provision was announced in 1985. This was the plan to replace the Resettlement Units, run by the (then) Department of Health and Social Security, by a range of smaller, less institutional accommodation, to be managed by local authorities or voluntary agencies.

During the 1980s, local authorities began to make greater use of low-quality bed and breakfast (B&B) hotels to accommodate the rising numbers of homeless people (Audit Commission 1989; Niner 1989). Soon, however, it became clear that the demand for accommodation for homeless people was not just a passing phenomenon, and the use of B&B hotels was resulting in a poor standard of service at a very high cost in many areas. Attempts were then made to reduce the use of B&B accommodation by diversifying into different types of temporary provision (such as private sector leasing, mobile homes, and 'homeless at home' policies) and by expanding the existing alternatives, such as hostels (Evans 1991).

Within the voluntary sector as a whole, the number of schemes providing housing with care and support grew dramatically during the 1980s. In 1980 there were 500, and by 1990 3,000, special needs schemes, developed by housing associations, often working in partnership with voluntary agencies (NFHA and SITRA 1991). Additionally, there was an expansion in the number of different groups of people accommodated. Thus, Watson and Cooper's study of supportive accommodation found that schemes established before 1970 provided for five groups, those established before 1980 for eight groups, and those before 1990 for fourteen groups (Watson and Cooper 1992). In contrast to the large shelters, many of the smaller hostels developed during the 1980s have fewer shared facilities and a more domestic atmosphere (Evans 1991). They usually offer better-quality accommodation than the more traditional hostels. Likewise, they provide more individual care and place a greater emphasis on recognising residents' needs for privacy and independence (Harrison *et al.* 1991).

As a result of such policies, hostels which conform to the traditional Victorian image now represent just a very small proportion of bed spaces and are by no means typical of the services available (Harrison *et al.* 1991). Rather, hostel provision in the 1990s is extremely diverse and consists of some high-quality as well as some low-quality accommodation. Indeed, supported housing now includes some accommodation which is no different from that provided by housing associations for single people generally, and some which differs significantly from mainstream provision. It therefore seems dangerous and inaccurate to cling to a simplistic belief that hostel accommodation is always and in all circumstances second-class and inferior. The aim of the next section is, however, to test such a hypothesis more rigorously by presenting some of the main findings from previous research.

EXISTING RESEARCH ON HOSTELS

There is already a vast amount of research into homelessness and provision for homeless people. This research includes reports by government departments, academic inquiries and studies by special interest or campaigning bodies. Whilst some research has considered hostels in their own right (for example, Garside *et al.* 1990), much important information about hostel provision can be obtained from studies which have a broader homelessness remit. Accordingly, a diverse range of reports are included in the discussion below.

Regarding the housing preferences of homeless people, one consistent finding arises from the existing literature. This is that the majority of homeless people desire their own independent and self-contained place – either a house, flat or bedsit (Drake *et al.* 1982; Garside *et al.* 1990; Smith *et al.* 1992; Anderson *et al.* 1993). There is, however, evidence to suggest that a minority of homeless people want or need more supported accommodation. Watson and Cooper, for example, found that a minority of people wanted long-term shared housing and these were likely to be older people who had previously lived in institutions (Watson and Cooper, 1992). Similarly, Garside *et al.* (1990) discovered that a preference for hostel accommodation was most frequently expressed by the older white residents who were currently living in provision with a high degree of staff cover. Cooper *et al.* (1993), meanwhile, concluded that sharing could provide particular benefits for some people who wanted security and informal support in addition to housing.

In terms of the evaluation of hostel accommodation itself, previous research has tended to focus on the more tangible and quantifiable aspects of provision. These have included funding (Berthoud and Casey 1988; Smith *et al.* 1991; Clapham *et al.* 1994); standards (physical conditions, location and design) (NACRO 1982; Garside *et al.* 1990; Evans 1991); the provision of support services and assistance with move-on (Berthoud and Casey 1988; Dant and Deacon 1989; Evans 1991); management and staffing (Garside *et al.* 1990; NFHA and SITRA 1991; Watson and Cooper 1992); and hostel policies and procedures (Garside *et al.* 1990; Smith *et al.* 1992). Some of the main findings relating to each of these topics are now considered below.

Funding

On the whole, studies have found that the mechanisms for funding hostel accommodation leave much room for improvement. For example, the limitations of revenue finance exert a strong influence on the design of supported housing by encouraging institutional accommodation in higher care schemes. Additionally, concern over the financing of schemes prevents the consideration or exploration of varied and imaginative 'packages' of care and support allowed for in the NHS and Community Care Act 1990 (Watson and Cooper 1992). In spite of such problems, research has, however, concluded that expenditure on hostels, which provide a half-way house between residential living and independence, is a worthwhile investment (Garside *et al.* 1990).

Standards: physical conditions, location and design

Some hostels occupy high-quality, purpose-built or fully converted premises with single rooms and plenty of facilities, and others have only unconverted properties, shared rooms and poor facilities. The hostels for the 'infirm' and for drug/alcohol abusers often have better than average premises, whilst women's refuges tend to have the worst (Berthoud and Casey 1988). According to NACRO (1982), the standard of a building, its physical condition, location and design are important factors which affect residents' self-esteem and say something about the way the project and the wider society perceive the inhabitants. Consequently, the provision of good-quality furniture and fittings is an important feature of hostel accommodation. It is, therefore, sensible to provide the minimum amount of good-quality, new or second-hand furniture that will stand up to the demands made of it. Similarly, noise and the use of communal space are potential sources of conflict and also warrant careful attention (NACRO 1982; Garside *et al.* 1990). Whilst smaller hostels are likely to be better for most people because they provided a useful step to independent living, for some they could be too difficult to adjust to, after living on the streets. For these people there might also be a need for larger hostels which can provide a degree of anonymity (Randall and Brown 1993).

Support services and assistance with move-on

The existing literature suggests that support services within hostels are haphazard, uncoordinated and in need of systematic review. The study by Berthoud and Casey (1988) concluded that some forms of support were provided for almost all the residents of almost all hostels, but this was only 'basic' or 'general' care. Garside *et al.* (1990) reported that client needs were seldom addressed and planned for directly and Evans (1991) found that the type of support/service provided in the hostels she studied depended on the skills and experience of key staff. According to Evans, this resulted in some offering little more than a caretaking service, whilst others offered intensive counselling on social/personal problems. Both Evans (1991) and Smith *et al.* (1992) highlighted the problems experienced by many hostel staff in dealing with a growing number of very vulnerable residents.

In terms of resettlement and move-on, research has concluded that, with the provision of appropriate support services (including financial support, as well as resettlement programmes for clients whilst in temporary accommodation, and outreach support once they have moved on), the level of successful resettlement of hostel residents could be improved (GLC/LBA 1981; Mullins 1991; Spaull and Rowe 1992). Nevertheless, some people might need or desire communal living. Likewise, there is a danger in over-emphasising the importance of settling in one place. A diversity of accommodation (including hostels) is consequently required. Moreover, there is also a need for a willingness amongst policy makers and service providers to recognise that what is effective as a home is different for different people according to their circumstances (Drake 1985; Tilt and Denford 1986; Dant and Deacon 1989; Walker *et al.* 1993).

Management and staffing

The arrangements for managing housing projects which offer support are very varied (Watson and Cooper 1992; Evans 1991). Likewise, there is considerable diversity in respect of the staffing arrangements. In their study of supported housing and housing associations, Watson and Cooper (1992) found that almost all schemes which opened before 1980 were managed directly by the association, whereas projects established in the early 1980s tended to be run in partnership with a voluntary agency or, less commonly, in conjunction with statutory agencies. In the study by Garside *et al.* (1990), the majority of hostels providing accommodation for single homeless people were voluntary organisations in partnership with housing associations. The type and number of staff for each hostel, meanwhile, tended to vary depending on the resources available, the needs of the residents and the aims of the hostel (Evans 1991).

Hostel policies and procedures

Garside *et al.* (1990) discovered that arrangements for referrals, acceptance policies and practices and intake procedures varied between hostels. Likewise, housing projects operated a range of policies regarding residents' rights of access to their accommodation (Harrison *et al.* 1991). In the past, many hostels limited the length of stay of homeless people, but as alternative sources of housing have grown increasingly scarce, time limits have frequently had to be reassessed and extended (Spaull and Rowe 1992). Rules and regulations are a common feature of almost all hostels. Nevertheless, exactly which ones are crucial, and how rigorously they should be enforced, is a moot point (Austerberry and Watson 1983; NACRO 1982). Given this wide variation in policies and practices, it is hardly surprising that research has consistently argued that inter-agency co-ordination and clear hostel aims and objectives are essential in order to ensure a coherent, efficient and effective approach to service delivery (Drake and Biebuych 1977; Drake *et al.* 1982; Jones 1987; Garside *et al.* 1990; McIvor and Taylor, 1995).

To summarise this section, the hostel sector comprises a very diverse range of provision and, although frequently inadequately and insufficiently funded, can and does provide a very valuable form of accommodation. Although hostels are not the preferred form of accommodation for the majority of homeless people, they do meet the needs and preferences of a minority. Moreover, even if hostel accommodation is not the preferred option of the majority of homeless people, it might be all that many are offered.

Existing research has produced a wealth of very detailed factual information about hostel accommodation and suggested various ways of improving it. Such information and recommendations are, however, largely of a quantitative nature and mostly relate to the more tangible aspects of provision (for example, funding, standards, support services, management, staffing, policies and procedures). To date little is known about the more conceptual and experiential aspects of hostel life. How, for example, do individuals feel about supported hostel accommodation? Is their quality of life improved because of it? Are they more or less independent after living there? To what extent do they sense that they have rights, control and choice? Or do they rather feel stigmatised, disempowered and excluded? These appear to be important questions also deserving of attention.

Additionally, existing evaluations of hostels have largely considered provision only from the perspective of providers (usually local authorities). Much less is known about supported accommodation from the perspectives of other relevant groups of individuals, such as residents, ex-residents, workers, management committee members, other involved professionals and the friends and relatives of residents. It is to such absent issues that the research discussed in the next section of this chapter addressed itself. This research, conducted during the spring and summer of 1994, formed the basis of a DPhil. thesis, completed by the present author in 1995 (Neale 1995).

HOSTELS REAPPRAISED

The research on which this section is based allowed individuals with direct experience of hostel accommodation to speak for themselves and to describe hostel life in their own words. In the process, a wide variety of topics were considered. These included both the more tangible and quantifiable features of provision discussed by earlier research (such as funding, standards and the availability of support services) as well as the more qualitative experiential aspects of hostel life (such as what it involves, how it feels, and what it means to live in a supported hostel for homeless people). In so doing, the study provided some useful insights into a range of topics which have hitherto received little attention from previous research. Examples of this included the role and relevance of hostel relationships; hostel atmosphere; stigma; dependence and independence; residents' feelings and emotions; and resident control, participation and choice.

Methods

A metropolitan city, which provided a broad range of supported hostel accommodation for homeless people, was selected as a case-study area. Four case-study hostels (A, B, C and D), chosen to reflect the diversity of provision in the city, were then used for further in-depth investigation. The research comprised forty-eight semi-structured interviews (twelve in each of the hostels), conducted with a mixture of residents, ex-residents, workers, managers, management committee members, referral agency representatives, volunteers and others.[1]

Hostel A was a large hostel (104 bedspaces) provided by a religious organisation for single men over 18 years of age. There was no maximum length of stay, beds were arranged in dormitories, and staff provided duty cover between 8 a.m. and 11 p.m. with an out-of-hours call system. *Hostel B* was a local authority hostel providing temporary accommodation for families. It had forty-six bedspaces arranged in different-sized living units with twenty-four-hour staff cover. *Hostel C* was a voluntary sector hostel offering accommodation and support, of indefinite duration, to single women over 30 years of age. Most residents had mental health needs which prevented them from coping in their own tenancies. The hostel had ten single bedspaces and provided office hours staffing with an out-of-hours call. *Hostel D* was part of a Christian organisation and offered accommodation to single homeless men aged 16–25 years. There was no minimum or maximum length of stay, as a result of which some of the current residents were older than 25. The hostel catered for any kind or level of need, providing eight single bedspaces and twenty-four-hour staff cover.

Findings

The research concluded that relationships were a fundamentally important aspect of hostel life. All respondent groups across all hostels reported that residents interacted in a mixture of ways, as in any living environment, but frequent quarrels were distressing. Many residents felt that the hostel was 'a home in part' or that they were 'a bit homeless'. Some residents considered the hostel to be their home, but also thought of themselves as homeless. Others did not consider themselves as homeless, but did not think of the hostel as home. In this way, the ambiguity and complexity of the meaning of home and homelessness (as discussed, for example, by Watson and Austerberry 1986; Gurney 1990; and Somerville 1992) were revealed.

Most respondents emphasised that whether or not residents considered the hostel to be home or themselves to be homeless depended upon the individual concerned, the particular hostel and its atmosphere, and individual interpretations of the meaning of 'home' and 'homelessness'. Feeling at home seemed to increase where residents had some choice about being in the hostel; felt secure, comfortable, and as though they belonged; had a degree of freedom and control over their daily living environment; were accommodated on a permanent, rather than a short-term basis; and had established some good inter-personal relationships.

Residents and non-residents argued that biased, negative, outdated stereotypical images of hostels, hostel residents and homeless people were the most likely causes of stigma. Although stigma was reported to be very difficult to challenge, some suggestions were advanced as to how it might be possible to begin to redress entrenched negative views. These included avoiding the word 'hostel', publicising the reasons why people become homeless, and remembering to treat residents as diverse individuals rather than as all the same.

Whilst both the residents and non-residents from all four hostels maintained that supported hostel accommodation was more likely to promote than to reduce independence, the ambiguity and complexity surrounding issues of dependence and independence were frequently recognised. Both residents and non-residents stressed that whether or not hostels increased or decreased independence depended on the particular hostel concerned and on the individual. Individual factors included residents' backgrounds, their mental and physical health, their support needs and their previous housing circumstances.

Across all four hostels and all respondent groups, the provision of help and support, safety and security, and assistance with move-on were considered to be the most valuable aspects of the accommodation. Greater practical assistance, changes to the management and to the general running of the accommodation, better building and facilities, increased funding and more effective inter-agency work were identified as the main potential improvements.

The characteristics most commonly highlighted as important by all respondents were the standards and the design (cleanliness, security, privacy and non-institutionalised appearance) and relationships (particularly staff–resident relationships). Hostel policies and procedures (rules, length of stay and daily routine); support services (day-to-day support and move-on); location (local facilities and proximity to town); and hostel atmosphere (that the environment was welcoming, happy, relaxed and homely) were also felt important by both the residents and the non-residents. Some staff, managers and other professionals additionally highlighted the relevance of resident participation, control and choice; clear hostel aims, objectives and philosophy; the availability of reliable funding; the provision of services which were flexible to individual requirements; the need to ensure that hostel costs did not make it difficult for residents to take up paid employment; and the need to reduce stigma.

Because the four case studies were catering for very different resident groups, it was difficult to compare the relative success of each in meeting residents' needs. *Hostel D* was, however, consistently evaluated the most positively by its residents and *Hostel C* the most negatively. *Hostel A* appeared to be meeting the needs of the older, but not the younger, residents, whilst *Hostel B* was essentially only catering for those requiring minimal support.

Given that the resources and the financial circumstances of each of the hostels were constrained, other reasons seemed to account for these different relative performances. The most probable explanation emerging from the research was the attention which each organisation afforded to a range of non-resource-dependent factors. These included good communication within and outside the organisation (especially effective inter-agency working); good manager–worker relations (particularly management support of staff); opportunities for resident choice; minimum paper work and bureaucracy; maximum individualised work with the residents; clear but flexible policies, procedures, aims and objectives; and a good hostel atmosphere.

Thus, *Hostel D* had invested much time and energy in developing and improving the running and the management of the accommodation; emphasised the value of good communication within and outside the organisation; had recently made efforts to increase its inter-agency work; recognised the need for consistent, but flexible, organisational aims, objectives and policies; and stressed the importance of the hostel environment and atmosphere. *Hostel C*, conversely, revealed an inability to respond to its changing resident population, exhibited confused management practices, poor relationships within the organisation and between the hostel and external bodies, unclear aims and objectives, and inconsistent policies and practices.

CONCLUSION

This chapter set out to question the role of hostels as a policy and practice response to homelessness. It found that provision varies enormously, both in type and in standards. Hostels may not be the preferred form of housing for the majority of individuals, but they do meet the needs of a minority. Significant improvements to existing provision are, however, both possible and desirable, and for this increased financial input is often, but not always, required. Many improvements can be made simply by placing a greater emphasis on the more experiential and conceptual aspects of hostel life. Examples of this would include promoting more supportive relationships; taking greater account of residents' feelings and emotions; creating a more pleasant hostel atmosphere; encouraging resident independence; confronting stigma; and increasing the opportunity for resident control, participation and choice. Indeed, as the third section highlighted, these more qualitative aspects of provision are as important as, and often inseparable from, the more material and quantifiable features.

To summarise, there is a need to challenge negative stereotypes about hostel accommodation and to reappraise provision more positively. This will, however, require evaluating both the qualitative and experiential aspects of hostel living (such as how it feels and what it means to live in a hostel), as well as the more quantitative and tangible features of provision (such as funding, standards, location and design). Likewise, it will involve evaluating provision from the perspectives of various interest groups and individuals (for example, residents, workers and other involved professionals, as well as providers).

Hostels are an important element in a coherent and effective strategy for tackling homelessness. They are not always a second-best alternative to other, more individualised living arrangements. Indeed, for some individuals, at some times in their lives, and for others more permanently, they can be a very valuable form of accommodation. Accordingly, hostels should not simply be used as an easy stop-gap for an inadequate housing market. Rather, they require sufficient financial investment, careful planning, skilful management and more appropriate methods of monitoring and evaluating their effectiveness.

NOTES

1 In the analysis, the opinions of all interviewees were examined. The expression 'residents' was used to refer to the 23 residents and the 4 ex-residents interviewed. The expression 'non-residents' was a collective term used to refer to the 8 workers, 1 relief worker, 3 managers, 2 management committee members, 1 volunteer, 3 referral agency representatives, 1 adult education tutor, 1 health visitor, and 1 community psychiatric nurse interviewed.

Chapter 15

Addressing the problem of youth homelessness and unemployment
The contribution of foyers

Deborah Quilgars and Isobel Anderson

Based on a French model, foyers are a relatively new model of supported accommodation for young people which have been developed
over the last five years in Britain. They differ from the majority of
previously existing hostels and supported housing for young people
by attempting to offer both temporary accommodation *and* training-
and employment-related services to residents (as well as sometimes
to non-residents). In the early 1980s, it was recognised that young
people were often finding it difficult to find a job because they lacked
an address, and similarly found it problematic trying to secure and
maintain good-quality housing whilst unemployed. Foyers were one
of a number of initiatives designed to address this 'no home, no job,
no home' catch-22 situation. This chapter examines this new form of
provision, and considers how successful foyers have been in meeting
the housing and employment needs of young people. The chapter
begins by discussing the nature of youth homelessness in the 1990s,
before looking at the introduction of foyers to Britain and presenting
the findings from an evaluation of a pilot scheme of foyers.[1] The
chapter ends by reflecting on the role of foyers, five years on from
their introduction to Britain.

YOUTH HOMELESSNESS IN BRITAIN IN THE 1990s

Young people are more likely to experience homelessness than any
other age group in the population (see Burrows, this volume). The
last Department of the Environment study of single homelessness
(Anderson *et al.* 1993) found that young people aged between 16
and 24 were considerably over-represented amongst single homeless
people, accounting for 30 per cent of people living in hostels and
bed and breakfast (B&B) establishments. As with homelessness

generally, it is accepted that youth homelessness grew significantly during the late 1980s and early 1990s, and that the problem affects all regions of Britain and both urban and rural areas. The recent inquiry into the prevention of youth homelessness (Evans 1996), set up to examine the escalating problem, estimated that approximately 246,000 young single people were homeless in the United Kingdom in 1995.

The reasons for this high level of youth homelessness are varied and complex. Most commentators identify a range of social and economic structural factors which have directly contributed to the rise in youth homelessness: in particular, changes to housing policy, the labour market and the benefit system (Hutson and Liddiard 1994; Carlen 1996; Evans 1996). Although the government has adopted a more individualised explanation of the causes of youth homelessness by suggesting that young people leave home too early, available evidence strongly indicates that many young people have no choice but to leave home (or the care system), and that young people do not choose to be homeless (Evans 1996). Jones's work on housing careers (1995) identifies how young people face differing levels of *risk* of experiencing homelessness depending on their market position (due to structural factors) and their individual strategies of survival. Young people who have little support or are unprepared for leaving home face the greatest risk of becoming homeless (Evans 1996).

It is no coincidence that the increase in youth homelessness has occurred over a period of time when 'normal' transitions from youth to adulthood have changed irrevocably. Coles (1995) and Jones (1995) identify three main transitions which young people typically experience: school to work; domestic transition from family of origin to destination; and housing transition from parental home to living independently. However, the traditional routes whereby people achieved the transition from childhood to adult life in the post-war years have been severely disrupted (Coles 1995; Roberts 1995; Jones 1995). Coles argues that these three transitions are now more complex, take longer and are more difficult to achieve successfully, resulting in many young people experiencing 'extended' or 'fractured' transitions. Changes in youth labour markets have been a particular cause for concern, with the 1991 Census demonstrating that the incidence of unemployment amongst 16–19-year-olds was twice that for the adult population as a whole (OPCS 1994). For those young people in employment, wages are low, and for those not in work, benefits are less than for the adult population aged 25 or over. Jones has also demonstrated how some young people now spend increasing periods of time in 'intermediate' housing, like hostels, lodgings or shared housing, as they are unable to access the reduced supply of social housing or enter owner occupation. Welfare provision has been cut at a time when unemployment has risen, with young people being disproportionately affected (Carlen 1996). This has made it much more difficult for young people to achieve smoothly the transition from a state of dependency to independence.

By the early 1990s, there was a broad acknowledgement of the close association between homelessness and unemployment, and how young people were disproportionately affected by both these social processes. This problem was commonly referred to as a cycle of 'no home, no job, no home'. Foyers were developed as one of a number of initiatives designed to help young people break out of this cycle by advocating an integrated approach to tackling both housing and employment needs. They were also seen as a possible way of easing the resultant difficult transition from youth to adulthood that young people were having to negotiate at a time of few jobs and reduced welfare protection (Shelter 1992).

THE INTRODUCTION OF FOYERS TO BRITAIN

The French foyer system was brought to the attention of the British housing world in 1991 by the housing campaign organisation Shelter. Concerned about the incidence of street homelessness amongst young people in Britain, Shelter sought to establish whether a similar problem existed in other European Union countries. Shelter's investigations suggested that youth homelessness was less evident in France compared to Britain, and that the network of *foyers pour jeunes travailleurs* (foyers for young workers) may have helped to prevent the escalation of homelessness during times of high unemployment (Shelter 1992).

There are approximately 450 foyers for young people in France, providing over 45,000 bedspaces. About half of the existing *foyers pour jeunes travailleurs* were established in France during the 1950s at a time of post-war industrial regeneration, with the aim of enabling young people to move to areas where there were shortages of labour. The other half were set up in the 1960s at a time of housing shortage but high unemployment rates. Expansion of the foyer network was financially supported by the French central government. A basic objective of many foyers was to provide young people with the necessary support to enable them to integrate into society as adults. Foyers in

France were primarily developed as a housing resource. However, in the 1980s as unemployment rose in France, and related to a modernisation programme of the existing foyers, they increasingly provided a role in helping young people train and find employment. It was this latter model of French foyers which was imported into Britain.

Shelter played a key role in campaigning for the development of foyers in Britain. A number of other agencies, mainly from within the voluntary housing movement, also became involved quite early on in the promotion of the idea of foyers. They included two large housing associations, London and Quadrant Housing Trust (L&QHT) and North British Housing Association (NBHA), the National Council of YMCAs and the Grand Metropolitan Trust. A considerable amount of lobbying took place to try to promote the idea of foyers. Approaches were made to government agencies, civil servants and politicians – including ministers and secretaries of state. A reflection of the success of this early lobbying was the fact that the then government included a commitment to piloting the foyer concept in its 1992 election manifesto.

The idea of developing a pilot programme of foyers came in large part from the Housing Corporation. The Housing Corporation had been approached by L&QHT and NBHA to provide capital funding to build two foyers. Whilst supporting these bids, the Corporation was concerned about the long lead-in time for construction of the purpose-built foyers, and advocated that the employment and training support services be piloted in existing hostels. YMCA (Young Men's Christian Association) hostels were chosen as a suitable testing vehicle, as they were considered to resemble French foyers most closely. The Employment Service (ES), part of the then Employment Department Group, agreed to the secondment of a key worker to L&QHT in order to develop the employment training and support services for pilot foyers. The pilot programme ran from 1992 to 1994 and is described on p. 220.

The pilot programme, however, was not the only feature of the early days of the foyer movement. As early as 1992, a momentum already existed for the development of foyers in Britain. The Housing Corporation, along with Shelter and the Architecture Foundation, set up a competition to build a foyer which offered a £1 million price (awarded to the then Shape HA). Also in 1992, a Foyer Federation for Youth (FFY) was set up by Shelter and Grand Metropolitan Trust to serve as an umbrella organisation to promote the development of foyers in Britain.

From the outset there was considerable support for the development of foyers from a diverse range of agencies. The initiative was perhaps unusual in attracting support from both campaigning organisations, like Shelter and other voluntary sector organisations, as well as the government, governmental organisations and the private sector. None the less, despite this consensus across different sectors, the foyer initiative was firmly challenged by some parts of the housing/voluntary movement (see Chatrik 1994 and housing press). The foyer concept as explained by its proponents did advance some controversial ideas. For example, foyers would offer general needs provision giving accommodation and support to a wide range of young people and not just to homeless, vulnerable applicants (Shelter 1992). Replicating the French model, foyers were anticipated to offer a large number of bedspaces, rather than the accepted wisdom of smaller units (Shelter 1992). It was also intended that foyers would somehow *link* accommodation to participation in job search or training for a job, an element that the government particularly stressed in their manifesto. As well as being controversial, the foyer concept also proved difficult to define precisely, with different parties attributing different qualities to foyers. This partly reflected the lack of information that was available on the French system.

In 1993, the FFY offered the following definition of a foyer: an integrated approach to meeting the needs of young people during their transition from dependence to independence by linking affordable accommodation to training and employment. It includes the following key elements: a target group of 16–25-year-olds; affordable, good-quality accommodation within a non-institutional framework; vocational training and jobs access support to residents; access to leisure and recreational facilities; a safe and secure environment; support and stability; and being part of a network in the United Kingdom and Europe. The pilot programme of foyers provided an opportunity for some of the emerging ideas regarding foyers to be tested.

THE EXPERIENCE OF THE PILOT FOYERS

The official pilot programme of foyers consisted of five existing YMCA hostels which converted to foyers (located in Nottingham, Norwich, St Helens, Wimbledon and Romford), and the two new-build schemes being developed by L&QHT and NBHA (in Camberwell, London, and Salford respectively). The YMCAs all became operational as foyers during 1992. The Camberwell foyer, managed by Centrepoint, was opened in November 1994, whilst the Salford foyer opened in January 1996 to be run by the YWCA. A two-year evaluation of the pilot programme of foyers in England was undertaken by the Centre for Housing Policy at the University of York, funded by the Joseph Rowntree Foundation (Anderson and Quilgars 1995). This chapter focuses on the operation of the five YMCA foyers.

The transition from a YMCA hostel to a foyer

The YMCAs were offering many of the key elements of a foyer as defined by the FFY definition prior to 1992. Most were already providing good-quality temporary accommodation, access to leisure and recreational activities and a safe and secure supportive environment. The main element which they needed to develop to become a foyer was vocational training and jobs access support to residents, in order to be able to offer an integrated approach to meeting young people's needs.

Employment and training support services were set up in the five YMCA foyers, usually consisting of a resource room staffed by two training/job search specialists. Facilities were provided such as computers, telephones, job vacancy boards and stationery. Revenue for the service was provided from two main sources: the then Employment Service Programme Development Fund and the Training and Enterprise Council Local Initiative Fund. Both of these funding sources were later to be incorporated into the Single Regeneration Budget. In the case of two foyers, Nottingham and St Helens, the local Employment Services office seconded a staff member to the foyer.

The employment and training support services offered similar services to that of a traditional Jobclub. However the services were delivered by a much less structured method. The resource area was typically operated as a drop-in facility rather than services being delivered as a course with a prescribed start and end date. Staff were also able to provide more intensive supervision to young people which covered a broader area than straightforward job search and training information. Considerable emphasis was placed on developing people's confidence and self-esteem, as well as generally supporting people and helping them address personal issues.

A detailed framework for referring young people to the foyer and delivering the foyer support services was devised by the Employment Services secondee to L&QHT. The model framework envisaged that applicants to the YMCA foyer would be jointly assessed by both existing housing management YMCA staff and the new employment/training support staff. Once accepted, an action plan would then be drawn up by the young person with the foyer worker, whereby the young person would outline his or her employment aims, and to a lesser extent housing aims. It was intended that this action plan would act as a contract outlining the young person's responsibilities to follow the action plan, revising it as necessary. The foyer support services would then support people in carrying out these aims by arranging training or work experience, assisting with job search and so on.

The YMCA foyers experienced difficulties in trying to put some of these elements of the framework into practice. The foyer support services were put into place with relative ease (despite some problems with locating the resource room), and staff were quite quickly in a position to assist young people with their employment aims. However, it proved more difficult to integrate these services into the existing YMCA operational procedures. In three YMCAs (and a fourth until very late in the pilot), the allocation procedure for the accommodation remained separate to the assessment for foyer employment and training services. Thus, housing staff assessed and accepted people into the hostel on the basis of housing need as before. When resident, the young person was then referred to the employment and training services if they were unemployed. The reasons for this appeared to be twofold: first, established staff were resistant to changing existing working practices in large part as they had not been consulted about the changes to the nature of the hostel; and second, some staff felt quite strongly as a matter of principle that access to the accommodation should not be conditional upon a young person's agreeing to use the employment and training services. In effect, only one pilot foyer explicitly tied residence in the hostel to use of the services.

The transition from YMCA to YMCA foyer was therefore not total in most of the YMCAs. The pilot experience showed how difficult it was to transform the culture of an existing hostel without implementing a total programme of staff training and reorientation, and how some foyer principles might conflict with existing priorities and aims. However, significantly, the pilot experience indicated that a fully integrated foyer operation (with joint assessment and a contract) was not a prerequisite for the successful operation of the foyer support services. Interestingly, the two least integrated hostels had very high levels of user satisfaction, with one achieving the highest level of success in placing people into jobs.

Who used the YMCA foyer services?

In the first eighteen months of the operation of the YMCA foyers, 500 people used the foyer employment and training services. As the referral and allocation procedures to the YMCA foyers had remained very similar, the client group reflected that of the existing YMCA. Three-quarters of those using the foyer support services were between the ages of 16 and 25 (with 7 per cent being 16–17), the official FFY age range for a foyer. A quarter of clients were over the age of 25, which largely reflected the YMCA policy of providing accommodation to 18–30-year-olds. Over four-fifths of foyer participants were male, which again reflected the overall higher number of men resident in the YMCAs. Nine out of ten participants were of a white ethnic origin.

The evaluation showed that the foyer participants were quite a vulnerable or disadvantaged group of young people (Table 15.1). This was not surprising, as the YMCAs taking part in the pilot had been operating either entirely or to a significant extent as 'special needs' hostels; that is, they were accommodating many young people who needed a range of support and assistance over and above the need for accommodation. A significant proportion of young people using the foyer support services had experience of the care system. As well as being in housing need at the point of entry into the foyer, nearly half of all foyer participants stated that they had slept rough at some time in the past. Over two-fifths of young people had been in trouble with the police at some time in

Table 15.1 Indicators of disadvantage

	% of foyer participants stating 'yes'
Past experience	
Lived in children's home	15
Lived with foster parents	9
Slept rough	47
Been 'in trouble' with the police	42
Present characteristics	
Long-term health problem affecting work	18
Difficulties with reading English	13
Difficulties with writing English	19
Difficulties with working with numbers	13

Source: Foyer Federation for Youth. Own analysis
Note:
Percentages do not sum to 100 per cent as more than one answer could be given

the past. A significant minority of clients reported a long-term (six months or more) health problem or disability which affected the type of paid work they could do, and a considerable minority had literacy and numeracy problems.

Measuring the success of the foyers

The pilot evaluation looked at a number of different measures of success, including data on the number of people who secured jobs and moved on to independent living, as well as more qualitative measures, through evaluating the value placed on the service by young people.

During the first eighteen months of the operation of the five foyers, 130 full-time jobs and 40 part-time jobs were found. Nearly 300 people engaged in job search, with more than 100 people undertaking a training programme. The funders of the support services, chiefly the Employment Service, were particularly interested in the extent to which young people were successfully placed into jobs and training. Although this level of success was lower than normal Jobclubs, the Employment Service appeared to be relatively encouraged by the pilot experience (Crook and Dalgleish 1994), as it was considered that many foyer clients were not ready to use a Jobclub, and therefore they were reaching a group of people that they might miss through more mainstream provision.

A quarter of people leaving the YMCA foyers left with both a job and permanent housing (83 people). Some people had worked whilst living in the YMCA but at the time of leaving were no longer working. The pilot experience showed that young people's lives did not necessarily follow a linear pattern of finding a job and then moving on into independent accommodation as envisaged in the original foyer framework. There were a variety of reasons why people left the YMCA foyer: for example, some found independent accommodation whilst they were still training; others left to go to college; and a considerable number had to leave due to a breach of their tenancy (unrelated to their search for employment). This last reason highlighted one of the disadvantages of providing employment and training services alongside accommodation services – when people left the foyer it proved very difficult to continue working with them as non-residents, especially when they had been evicted.

Whilst finding jobs and housing was the ultimate aim of the foyers, the evaluation of the foyer pilots showed that the process of providing support was just as important as the final outcome. Staff and users explained that for some people who had been unemployed for a long period of time and had a low self-esteem, success could mean having the confidence to go for an interview rather than actually securing the job. It was clear that the high level of take-up enjoyed by the foyer services was largely due to the flexible, client-centred way in which services were delivered. Most young people used the services without any compulsion, demonstrating that a contract linking participation to residence in the hostel was unnecessary. Users appreciated the support and respect offered to them by staff, and liked the fact that the service offered more than just help with training and employment. Many said that they preferred the foyer approach to more formal government programmes. Some clients felt that they had undertaken training, job search or employment which they would not have done without the help of the foyer, or would have done less intensively or with less enthusiasm.

> I don't think I would have got those three interviews if I hadn't been here. So this place has helped me quite a bit.
>
> (Foyer user)

> What I like about it, I mean they're not here to help you just find a job, or whatever, they do help you with your personal problems – it's nice to know that you're not here just for one thing, you can talk about whatever problems you have.
>
> (Foyer user)

> I just picked myself up and went for it. But I wouldn't have done it without their help.
>
> (Foyer user)

> The young people we've been able to help, obviously that's the main satisfaction . . . to actually see the changes in people means everything to me. They may not have a job but they are losing their aggression, developing a sense of responsibility, feeling more comfortable with themselves . . . . We try to make them feel that they've got something to offer. Sometimes they've tried work and maybe not lasted very long, but they've tried and they've got work, and it's going to be that much easier the next time.
>
> (Foyer worker)

The impact on youth homelessness and unemployment

The main success of the pilot YMCA foyers was in enabling disadvantaged young people to increase their confidence and compete more effectively for existing employment and housing opportunities. However, the foyers were not able to make any significant impact on wider socio-economic factors. Foyers were developing at a time of recession in Britain and, although they were successful in establishing some links with employers, and beginning to change local employer attitudes to homeless young people, they could not change the fact that most employers had few vacancies and most commonly offered temporary and low-paid work. Similarly, whilst the YMCAs were providing a valuable accommodation resource to young people, they were constrained in their attempts to help people to move on by the wider housing market and the general shortage of local affordable accommodation for young single people. The new-build pilot foyers offer new additional bedspaces to young people but they face the same problems in trying to find appropriate secure accommodation for people leaving the foyer. The new-build foyers also experienced significant problems in finding the necessary capital to build the foyer, indicating that replication of the model on a large scale would be difficult.

The experience of the pilot foyers provided further confirmation that the transition from youth to adulthood was not straightforward or necessarily linear in nature. Finding full-time permanent jobs, with secure housing, proved elusive for many foyer participants. The YMCA foyers were pro-active in encouraging people to explore a range of alternatives, from training to education, as well as broader life experiences like taking part in Raleigh International. The pilot experience indicated that foyers *needed* to take this broader approach in order to support young people's creative efforts to make the difficult transition from youth to adulthood in the 1990s.

FOYERS: FIVE YEARS ON FROM THEIR INTRODUCTION TO BRITAIN

Many commentators thought that foyers were the 'flavour of the month' when they first arrived in Britain, and asserted that they would not survive their high-profile and controversial entrance to the housing world. However, despite such speculations, the support for foyers does not appear to have waned and the development of foyers has proceeded at a steady pace over the last five years. Whilst the target of Shelter and the FFY of developing between 200 and 500 foyers in Britain by the year 2000 (Shelter 1992) is unlikely to be reached, it is possible that there will be approximately 100 foyers by the end of the century. This would represent quite a significant achievement given the difficulties with securing funding experienced by the pilot agencies, though it should be noted that a good number of these would be converted hostels rather than new-build foyers.

By the end of 1996, there were forty-five operational foyers, with thirty-eight in development and twenty-nine foyers planned (see Table 15.2). The vast majority of the foyers were in England, with only two foyers in Scotland and none in Wales. Nearly two-thirds of the existing foyers were located in urban areas and over a third in rural settings. Within England, the foyers were fairly evenly spread throughout the country. Should this pattern of development continue it is possible that an effective network of foyers could exist in Britain by the year 2000. However, this would require the development of systems so that young people wishing to move from one foyer to another could do so. This could be difficult to achieve, as foyers would need to operate compatible referral and allocation procedures.

The present foyer movement is characterised by a diversity of provision. It is clear that foyers have developed to a variety of different models. Whereas the original model of a foyer was seen as a large building, which to be economically viable would need to provide between 50 and 80 beds, research has shown that foyers now range in size from 8 to 177 beds (Annabel Jackson Associates 1996). Foyers are also offering a range of different types of accommodation and services: some provide hostel-type bedrooms with shared facilities, whilst others offer shared flatlets, and others have opted for self-contained units. Dispersed models of foyers have also been developed, where accommodation is provided in shared houses

Table 15.2 Number of foyers in Great Britain

	No.	%
Operational foyers	45	
London	7	15
Other urban districts	22	49
Rural districts	16	36
Foyers in development	38	
Foyers planned	29	

Source: Foyer Federation for Youth, November 1996. Own analysis

around a town or city with the training and employment services also being delivered on a separate site. This diversity in foyer provision is likely to continue as agencies respond to young people's needs at a local level.

A lack of information still exists on some aspects of foyer work. Although some foyers are clearly catering for a more vulnerable group of young people than others, the precise client group for foyers remains ill-defined and open to debate. Given the enduring problem of homelessness amongst young people, it is likely that most foyers will provide accommodation to a significant proportion of vulnerable young people. However, schemes could run into problems if they are designed to offer minimal support and then need to cater for people with high support needs. The issue of whether accommodation should be tied to participation to a foyer programme seems to have fallen down the agenda, and at present it is unclear how many foyers are operating to this principle and to what effect. It is also unclear how the new housing benefit changes affecting young people will impact on foyers – demand may go up as a result of young people finding it more difficult to find affordable self-contained accommodation.

Foyers are likely to continue to exist and develop, at least in the medium-term future. The introduction of foyers to Britain has served to draw attention to the difficult problems that young people face in finding housing and employment in the 1990s. However, one needs to be realistic about the contribution that foyers can make to addressing youth homelessness and unemployment. They may be a valuable addition to the range of provision which is on offer to homeless young people, but they do not eradicate the need for the search for more enduring solutions to the problem of youth homelessness in Britain.

NOTES

1   This evaluation was funded by the Joseph Rowntree Foundation and is more fully reported in Anderson and Quilgars (1995).

Chapter 16

Working together to help homeless people
An examination of inter-agency themes

Christine Oldman

Section 73 of the 1985 Housing Act (s.73) (now Section 180 of the 1996 Act) empowered the Secretary of State to give grant aid for the purposes of preventing and relieving homelessness. In the early 1990s the Department of the Environment's s.73 programme was concerned with assisting voluntary sector organisations working with single homeless people. The provision of services to people who are homeless inevitably involves agencies working with one another in different ways. Although there is a large academic literature on joint working, this is concerned, in the main, with relationships between health and social care organisations and has little to say about collaborative working involving housing agencies. The aim of this chapter is to examine the nature of joint working in the field of homelessness taking the s.73 programme as a case study. The chapter begins by discussing the policy context in which local homeless networks operate and then describes empirical work designed to evaluate the s.73 programme with respect to four major issues:[1] first, the extent to which projects went beyond their remit by working with *statutorily* homeless people; second, the extent to which projects went beyond their remit by addressing non-housing need; third, the manner in which the need for services was being demonstrated; and fourth, the degree to which there was developing unnecessary duplication of provision in local areas.

POLICY CONTEXT: HOMELESSNESS AND HOUSING STRATEGIES

In any local area a whole range of organisations are involved, in some way or other, in the purchasing or providing of services for homeless people. Elsewhere in this book the social construction of homelessness which results in the compartmentalising of homelessness into discrete categories such as *rough sleepers, single homeless* and *priority homeless* has been discussed. It will become evident in this chapter that this artificial splitting up of the 'homeless problem' determines how agencies work with one another to prevent or relieve homelessness.

The starting point of any investigation of joint working in the area of homelessness has to be the local authority housing department. As has been made very clear (Lowe, this volume), local authorities are only obliged to accommodate those families and single people who are in 'priority need'. They have, however, to provide 'appropriate advice and assistance' in finding accommodation for those homeless people who have not been categorised as being in priority need. Local authorities interpret this duty in a number of different ways. Some give minimal assistance, whilst others work actively with other local agencies, maintain accommodation registers and make accommodation available for non-priority homeless people. In their relatively new role of 'enabling', local authority housing departments have been increasingly encouraged by the Department of Environment (DoE) to develop single homeless strategies as part of their responsibility to assess housing need more generally. Such strategies must involve other agencies:

> Local authorities should aim to provide a strategic framework of assistance covering all the agencies involved in meeting the needs of the single homeless (including rough sleepers) within their area. The capacity for an authority to co-ordinate with social services department, and with outside agencies is vital.
>
> (Department of the Environment 1994b)

Local housing authorities, then, variously provide and/or fund services for priority and non-priority homeless people. In doing this they work with other agencies. As far as provision for non-priority homeless people is concerned, they work with the voluntary sector, funding development and revenue costs for housing schemes, funding resettlement and advice projects and referring clients. At the time of writing this chapter it is not possible to say what effect the changes to homelessness legislation contained within the 1996 Housing Act will have on joint working.

POLICY CONTEXT: COMMUNITY CARE AND HOMELESSNESS

It has been suggested above that housing departments have an incentive to work with non-housing agencies in order to address housing need. Equally, social and health care agencies have an incentive to work with housing organisations in order to address adequately the community care needs of their various clientele. Traditionally, homelessness and community care have been viewed as distinct areas – housing departments' priorities such as tackling homelessness took them away from working with other agencies in the field of community care. Recently, however, there has been a spate of policy guidance and research evidence which very firmly places housing and community care side by side. Indeed, the implementation of community care itself has, arguably, resulted in an increase in homelessness. A number of commentators (Shanks and Smith 1992; Scott 1993) have noted that the process of de-institutionalisation has brought with it an increase in the visibility of homeless people with mental health problems.

In the early days of the 'new' community care there was general criticism that the role of housing had been neglected (Oldman 1988; Means and Smith 1994). However, more recently progress, although slow, is being made in involving housing agencies in the community care planning process encouraged by a range of policy guidance. The 1992 DoE/DoH circular on community care stressed the need for inter-agency collaboration in relation to people with community care needs. In 1993 the Department of Health brought out guidance (DoH 1993) specifically on the links between homelessness and community care. It was acknowledged that homelessness was not simply a housing problem. Concern had been expressed that social services were focusing too much on *priority groups,* most notably older people. Prior to April 1993 housing projects had autonomy over the assessment of clients who were funded through the DSS residential allowance. With the abolition of that benefit, projects registered under the Residential Homes Act must turn to their local social service authorities for funding support. The Support Force paper (DoH 1993) urged social service departments to develop skills in managing what it called the social care market: 'The starting point is for Social Service Departments to accept that the community care needs of homeless individuals is an area for which they have responsibility and which needs managing' (DoH: 1993: 6).

The paper also urged housing authorities and social services to work together to resolve any difficulties over definitions of 'ordinary residence' and 'local connection'. In order to get housing, homeless people must prove a local connection. To obtain a social services assessment homeless people must be ordinarily resident in the area and 'vulnerable'. However, as Pinch (1993) notes, a social services authority can define vulnerability in a different way from its housing department. The Support Force paper urged housing and social service authorities to develop joint protocols for providing 'fast track' assessment and services. It condemned 'buck-passing'.

A year after the publication of the Support Force paper, the Department of Health's special monitoring study of the housing aspects of community care looked at how well inter-agency collaboration relating to homelessness was working in its ten sample local authorities. Particular issues it focused on were the role of inter-agency fora in developing a strategic view on overall provision, and the need for early inter-agency hospital discharge planning in order to avoid last-minute referrals or solutions.

As well as the Department of Health itself, other bodies have highlighted the need for agencies to co-operate in order to address the needs of homeless people. The Royal College of Physicians (Connelly and Crown 1994) concluded there was an urgent need for a wide-ranging national policy review of housing and community care policies. Within such a joint policy local authorities and health authorities should review current medical prioritisation procedures and integrate them with community care assessment procedures. The Standing Conference on Public Health (Knight 1994) also noted the adverse effect of inadequate housing on community care policies and, equally, the effect of inadequate care and support on the ability of people to sustain tenancies. It called for more progress to be made in involving homeless people themselves in the development and direction of services.

Considerable national attention has recently been paid to the problems of providing community care to severely mentally ill people:

> Time and time again, homeless people with mental health problems receive only short term help from psychiatric services, inadequate follow up and no improvement in their housing situation on discharge. It is a failure of joint working which is dangerous,

wasteful of resources and within the power of authorities to substantially and rapidly improve.

(Prior 1994)

A survey carried out by the NHS Advisory Service highlighted the uncoordinated approach to the commissioning and provision of services for homeless people and a House of Commons Committee criticised disputes over funding the government's Homeless Mentally Ill Initiative.

Increasingly, documentation is appearing concerning local initiatives across the country where attempts have been made to address the problems discussed above. For example, the London Borough of Islington has developed a client-focused model of assessment for community living. Homeless applicants are considered under the same assessment criteria as other residents in the borough and may refer themselves (Pinch 1993). Assessment is neighbourhood based and multidisciplinary to ensure effective local liaison with health and community services. Camden, too, has adopted a comprehensive approach, including a multi-agency panel which agrees common definitions of vulnerability (DoH 1994).

Obstacles to joint working

Despite all the recent exhortations to organisations to work together, key features of the community care reforms present formidable problems for joint working. The introduction of market principles, albeit in different forms in each of the three sectors – health, social care and housing – is a major obstacle. As Nocon views it:

Until now providers have been part of the planning process contributing considerable expertise about needs and ways of meeting them. But how can their continued input be reconciled with the market system when those providers may be beneficiaries of the purchasing process? An increasing amount of health authority business is already being conducted behind closed doors for reasons of commercial confidentiality; there is a real contradiction between the new ethos of competition and the call for collaboration.

(Nocon 1994: 28)

The newly established split between the purchasing and providing of services complicates and alters traditional methods of joint working. The number of 'interfaces', for example, has considerably increased, particularly since 1996 with the implementation of a purchaser–provider split in housing through the introduction of Compulsory Competitive Tendering (CCT) in housing management. Providers do not have an equal relationship with purchasers, and housing and social services with their dual role as providers and purchasers are in competition with other providers. However, commentators have argued that joint working in the 1990s may be more purposive than before: 'Within the new arrangements, the emphasis is on negotiation, bargaining, contracts, doing business together, performance, accountability and (in theory at least) outcomes for users rather than the more general and often unfocused joint planning of the past' (Nocon 1994: 28).

Working with other agencies

Other recent legislation has implications for services and provision for homeless people – namely, the Criminal Justice Act 1991 and the Children Act 1989. The 1991 Act, which introduced community sentencing and emphasised continuity of supervision in custody, reflects similar principles to the community care legislation. The DoH special monitoring study (1994) noted that social services departments were insufficiently linked with the criminal justice system and the Probation Service. The Children Act sets out a framework for services for care leavers and defines the provision to be made for young homeless people. The Act specifies that local authorities must provide appropriate accommodation and support for any young person aged 16 or 17 and 'in need'. Evaluation of the housing aspect of the Act's operation has revealed, however, that some local authorities are failing to meet the needs of 16- and 17-year-olds primarily because, as with community care, the inter-agency co-operation between housing and social services required to achieve joint assessment has not been fully developed (McCluskey 1993).

EVALUATION OF THE SECTION 73 GRANT PROGRAMME

At the time of the evaluation the section 73 grant programme was virtually the only central government commitment to non-statutory homelessness outside London. As already outlined, the purpose of the programme is to enable the voluntary sector to provide *services* for non-statutory homeless people (in contrast to the Rough Sleepers Initiative, which funds bricks and mortar provision as well as support

services). Although there is considerable variety in how s.73 projects
are constituted, they fall into two main types: accommodation registers and resettlement services – although there is no very clear distinction between the two. Accommodation register projects would
variously encourage landlords to let to homeless people, facilitate the
expansion of available rented accommodation and build up and maintain registers of appropriate accommodation usually in the private
rented sector (PRS). Resettlement projects typically help people,
who appear to have needs over and above the need for accommodation, to settle from the streets or hostel accommodation into more
permanent accommodation.

Methodology

An audit of provision for homeless people was carried out in six
areas. The areas were: a metropolitan district council; a large, non-
metropolitan district; a resort area comprising three district councils; a mixed urban and rural area comprising three district councils
within one shire county; a predominantly rural area comprising
three district councils within one shire county; and a predominantly
rural area comprising seven district councils in two shire counties.
The aim of the audit was to collect as much information as possible
about service planning and provision for homeless people, whether
deemed 'statutory' or otherwise. Telephone interviews were conducted first with the twenty-five s.73 projects operating in the areas
and then with other organisations, statutory and non-statutory,
named by the projects as being involved in homelessness. Each
organisation interviewed was asked to list all the organisations with
whom they had contacts. Finally, a picture of 'local homeless networks' was built up. In addition to collecting quantitative data about
provision and services, more qualitative information about the
effectiveness of joint working was sought. In total, eighty interviews were achieved.

Some findings

Working together within the housing sector

The key finding of the study was that there was extensive inter-
agency working in all the six areas between and within different
segments of the 'homelessness system', but that this mainly

concerned the process of client referrals. There was less evidence of a strategic or overall co-ordination of services delivery. As a result, in most of the areas, particularly in the urban centres, there were both major gaps in provision *at the same time* as a degree of overlap between services. Some individual schemes for homeless people in areas where a number of organisations had reported considerable unmet need had fairly high levels of voids.

The voluntary sector organisations worked closely with their local authority housing departments in terms of two-way referrals. The s.73 projects were funded to work with non-priority homeless people, but of the projects' client case load around a third were considered to be in priority need. The boundaries between the categories 'priority' and 'non-priority' are very blurred. Local authorities vary quite considerably in their interpretation of 'vulnerability' and hence whom they will accept and subsequently house (Butler *et al.* 1994). However, there were other reasons why s.73 projects worked with the 'priority homeless'. The projects were quite often the first point of access to services and accommodation for homeless people, and hence they provided a supportive role whilst clients' eligibility was being checked out. Some projects also provided a resettlement service only for people who had been accommodated under the provisions of the homelessness legislation in hostel or other temporary accommodation. The mechanics of joint working varied from area to area depending on the local authority's homelessness policies and practices. Some had a very active, direct role both towards priority and non-priority homeless, whilst others assumed a minimal role even towards those for whom they had a statutory responsibility contracting out resettlement and advice services to the voluntary sector.

Although relationships between voluntary sector organisations and the housing department were generally described as being good, there were many instances of dispute between the two over interpretations of homeless legislation. There were disagreements about the relative responsibilities of the housing authority and the voluntary sector. The voluntary sector organisations, because they were often in receipt of grant aid or were in a service agreement, felt that there was an imbalance of power which affected joint working.

Within and between sectors

A considerable amount of joint working was reported to be going on within the voluntary sector *and* with health and social care agencies over client referral and assessment. This type of joint working was viewed as largely beneficial: 'We don't just liaise with agencies but joint work with them. It's week in, week out, joint working. There's real communication between projects on individuals that is innovative because it increases the quality of the work and improves results and fast tracks people into services' (s.73 project manager).

Voluntary agencies referred clients to one another; relationships were, however, sometimes marred by competition over clients and resources. Nor was there necessarily complete knowledge concerning organisations' goals, practices and allocation procedures. Voluntary sector agencies often had difficulty obtaining health and social care services for their clients, and sometimes felt that the latter were referring clients to them whom they felt they were unable to help adequately: 'If someone is seen to have a very, very chaotic lifestyle or is unable to meet their own care needs, like have their own medication or feed themselves, then they have obviously got a very much higher need than we can deal with' (voluntary sector housing support worker).

Although, as the quotation above shows, agencies often did feel that they could not cope with certain 'special needs', they generally felt that demarcation disputes over what characterised joint working in the area of housing and community care were unhelpful. They were clear, however, that a simplistic separation as to what is a housing activity and what is not is impossible:

> Your basic need is food and drink and after that's met then there's shelter. And once that's met other needs begin to surface. And once they do start surfacing the irony is that it is housing that has enabled those needs to arise and the irony of it is that those needs arising can actually cause somebody to lose their housing because they can't actually deal with those issues and therefore everything goes. So the bills aren't paid, the rent isn't paid and so on. But you need the skills to actually help that person recognise what's happening to them and reflect back to their experience and that takes quite a lot of sophisticated skills. . . . It isn't quite as simple as saying that this is a housing thing and this is a support thing because in reality in all the work we do, if we simply said 'This is s.73 funding, all we are going to do is to advise them on housing benefit and service connections and see you next month' then it's a recipe for disaster. If you take a very simplistic division of this

is housing and this is support then again in practice that division is not actually there.

(s.73 project worker)

Voluntary sector organisations working with homeless people are set up on multidisciplinary grounds; they do not want to worry about which part of their work is housing and which not. However, the funding world they work in is compartmentalised on these lines.

In addition to these sort of problems there were a range of other difficulties surrounding joint working. Different agencies failed to understand how the others worked, and in particular there was often misunderstanding regarding the voluntary sector. Different professional perspectives also presented a problem. For example, there is a long history of enmity between housing and social service professionals in which negative stereotypes abound (BASW 1985). Some voluntary sector projects reported they were failing to get referrals from social services departments because the latter were not in sympathy with independent living ideals that projects believed they espoused.

Gaps and overlaps

The audit of provision revealed that there were significant gaps. In all the areas there was lack of appropriate 'move-on' accommodation, particularly supported accommodation, and a paucity of resettlement services to prevent tenancies failing. Interviews with clients also suggested there was a chronic shortage of services such as rent guarantee schemes and advice services to help homeless people access the PRS. At the same time, areas reported that there was considerable service overlap. The concept of overlap is not easy to define. It can mean either similarity or over-provision. Overlap in terms of similarity was frequently seen as both inevitable and appropriate: 'Yes, there's overlap but there's not over provision. Overlap is OK as it means we can refer a client to another organisation which may be better at dealing with someone' (local authority housing advice worker).

It was felt that it was very important to give users some choice and flexibility, but in some areas there was, arguably, a certain degree of *duplication* of provision. Such a state of affairs plays into the hands of resources-starved commissioning authorities and considerably weakens statements from bidding organisations concerning local unmet need. Different agencies were assuming different roles and providing different or similar services to different client groups, often in the absence of an explicitly co-ordinated policy towards provision for homeless people. Co-ordination, however, results in better information about services, which benefits both clients and providers and produces a better use of scarce resources. The research's interviews with clients showed that they found a lack of information on the range of services provided; a freephone line was suggested by one particular client.

Inter-agency fora

In some areas, progress towards better co-ordination was being made, and increasingly inter-agency homelessness fora were being set up. The fora varied quite considerably in terms of their member-ship, their terms of reference and their effectiveness. Some, for example, were loose coalitions of purchasers (housing, health and social services) and providers. The latter inevitably felt that purchasers' interests were dominant. A number of fora were involved in genuine co-ordinating activity: assessing local need, reviewing existing provision and developing plans for future service provision. The problems facing fora trying to develop homelessness strategies should not be underestimated. As other chapters of this book have shown, assessment of the incidence of homelessness and its charac-teristics is complex and difficult.

In a number of areas there were examples of centralised services, such as a clearing house for referrals or a centralised accommodation register which could be accessed by several agencies. However, there was not a great deal of support for collaborative service provision or joint bidding to funding organisations. There were concerns that 'rationalisation' of services would lead to a lack of diversity of users. Also it was felt that inter-agency working had become increasingly difficult in an environment of competition. Organisational survival was seen as a more important priority than the cost-effective use of resources, although it was recognised that joint application for fund-ing might in some circumstances secure continuation of an activity, albeit in a slimmed-down form.

SOME CONCLUSIONS

The evaluation showed that services for homeless people must address need in a holistic way. It also showed that the discrete parcelling up of homelessness into categories such as 'priority' and 'non-priority', 'special need' versus 'ordinary' homelessness, 'single' homelessness versus 'family' homelessness and so on impedes joint working and does a disservice to those people who are without secure accommodation. Strategic co-ordination of services was not much in evidence but the problems in achieving it are formidable. Finally, a general lack of resources, particularly of suitable, safe and well-supported housing, is a further impediment to successful joint working.

The s.73 evaluation was carried out in 1994 but its findings remain valid at the time of writing. Pleace's (1995; this volume) study of local authority services to priority single homeless people discussed elsewhere in this book graphically illustrates the problems of inadequate support for resettlement services from social service departments. Two of Pleace's respondents comment as follows:

> When we've made a referral to social services it can be anything up to six weeks before you get an actual acknowledgement. In the meantime this individual is becoming more and more dependent on the resettlement service support and if they should be lucky enough to get a support worker from social service the input isn't a great deal, we don't feel anyway.

> What you find with social services is the minute they find out there is a support worker involved, they think great, we can pull out.

(Pleace 1995:52)

Pleace (1995) recommends that joint assessment of statutorily homeless single people should be required by law. Pleace and Quilgars' (1996; this volume) review of health and homelessness in London confirms the s.73 finding relating to the issue of overlap. They found that the number of agencies which had some input into the broad welfare of homeless people numbered just under 200 and that no one central register of resources existed. Agencies were not even always aware of one another's existence.

In 1996 three chief executives of nationally known voluntary sector organisations got together to condemn the failures of the 'new' community care (Harker *et al.* 1996). Involved in the provision of accommodation and support for vulnerable and often homeless people they catalogued extensively endemic problem shunting and the revolving door syndrome. They concluded that the fundamental divisions that exist between and within sectors are not the result of poor communication or lack of experience of inter-agency working. Rather, they are due to structural and institutional barriers or fault lines.

Finally, although it did not look at homelessness in any great detail, a study appearing in late 1996 also confirmed the findings of the s.73 evaluation, arguing that:

> A competitive culture can lead to a narrow and specialist approach to services, discouraging inter agency working. The emphasis on making agencies more 'accountable' for their performance can also lead to a focus on narrow indicators which work against collaboration and the achievement of long-term goals.
>
> (Joseph Rowntree Foundation 1996)

Previous empirical studies of joint working have tended not to focus particularly on inter-agency collaboration concerning homelessness. This chapter has examined the nature and extent of joint working, both within sectors and between sectors, in this area. It has shown the central importance of housing and support services and provision for homeless people to the successful implementation of community care policies and practices. The s.73 projects had a fair degree of success preventing and relieving homelessness and they had a better record of involving users in the assessment and delivery processes than some of their other partners. There were, however, significant problems around joint working.

Due, in part, to a lack of strategic co-ordination of service delivery, there are significant gaps in provision at the same time as a situation of overlap of both services and provision. However, it is no surprise at all that joint working is imperfect. To borrow from Adrian Webb's famous phrase, joint working failures have littered the policy landscape from the time of Poor Law reform onwards. Agencies are reluctant to give up the freedom and independence that joint working means unless they can very clearly see the benefits. The 'new' community care is inherently contradictory. On the one hand, agencies are exhorted to get together but, on the other, competition between organisations has been built into the reforms. Homelessness presents particular problems for joint working; assessing need and delivering health and social care services to an itinerant population is immensely difficult. A serious lack of resources particularly, relating to appropriate housing and its concomitant support services, continues to be a major obstacle. There are further difficulties coming along. Finally, inter-agency disputes are not only between housing, health and social care organisations. The Department of Social Security is also involved. Increasingly the DSS is adopting a particularly narrow definition of what is a housing cost. This policy drift threatens a whole range of housing and support provisions which depend very largely on housing benefit for their survival (Oldman *et al.* 1996).

NOTES

1   This evaluation was funded by the Department of the Environment (DoE 1995b). The views expressed in this chapter are those of the author and are not necessarily those of the DoE.

References

Adamczuk, H. (1992) *Sleeping Rough in Birmingham*, Birmingham: Birmingham City Council.

Anderson, I. (1993) 'Housing policy and street homelessness in Britain', *Housing Studies* 8(1):17–28.

—— (1994) *Access to Housing for Low Income Single People*, York: Centre for Housing Policy, University of York.

Anderson, I., Kemp, P. and Quilgars, D. (1993) *Single Homeless People*, London: HMSO.

Anderson, I. and Quilgars, D. (1995) *Foyers for Young People: Evaluation of a Pilot Initiative*, Centre for Housing Policy, University of York.

Annabel Jackson Associates (1996) *Foyers: The Step in the Right Direction*, London: Foyer Federation for Youth.

Arblaster, L., Conway, J., Foreman, A. and Hawtin, M. (1996) *Setting us up to Fail: a Study of Inter Agency Working to Address Housing, Health and Social Care Needs of People in General Needs Housing*, Bristol: Policy Press.

Audit Commission (1989) *Housing the Homeless: the Local Authority Role*, London: HMSO.

—— (1994) *Finding a Place: A Review of Mental Health Services*, London: HMSO.

Austerberry, H. and Watson, S. (1983) *Women on the Margins: a Study of Single Women's Housing Problems*, City University, London: Housing Research Group.

Bailey, R. (1992) 'No deposit, no return', *Inside Housing* (21 Aug.).

Banion, M. and Stubbs, C. (1986) 'Rethinking the terms of tenure: a feminist critique of Mike Ball', *Capital and Class* 29, (Summer): 182–94.

Banks, C. and Fairhead, S. (1976) *The Petty Short-term Prisoner*, Chichester: Barry Rose.

Barrett, M. and McIntosh, M. (1982) *The Anti-social Family*, London: Verso.

Barrett, M. and Phillips, A. (eds) (1992) *Destabilizing Theory: Contemporary Feminist Debates*, Cambridge: Polity Press in association with Blackwell Publishers, Oxford.

Barry, A.M., Carr-Hill, R. and Glanville, J. (1991) *Homelessness and Ill Health: What Do We Know? What Should be Done?* York: Centre for Health Economics, University of York.

Basuk, E.L. (1984) 'The homelessness problem' *Scientific American,* 251: 28–33.

Bayliss, E. and Logan, P. (1987) *Primary Health Care for Homeless Single People in London: a Strategic Approach,* London: Single Homeless in London Health Group.

Beck, U. and Beck-Gernsheim, E. (1996) 'Individualization and "precarious freedoms": perspectives and controversies of a subject-orientated sociology', in P. Heelas, S. Lash and P. Morris (eds), *Detraditionalization,* London: Blackwell.

Beevor, A. (1990) *Inside the British Army,* London: Corgi.

Berthoud, R. and Casey, B. (1988) *The Cost of Care in Hostels,* Research Report 680, London: Policy Studies Institute.

Berthoud, R. and Kempson, E. (1992) *Credit and Debt: the PSI Report,* London: PSI.

Best, S. and Kellner, D. (1991) *Postmodern Theory: Critical Interrogations,* New York: The Guilford Press.

Bevan, M., Kemp, P. and Rhodes, D. (1995) *Private Landlords and Housing Benefit,* Research Report, University of York.

Bevan, M. and Rhodes, D. (1997) *Can the Private Rented Sector House the Homeless?* York: Centre for Housing Policy.

Bines, W. (1994) *The Health of Single Homeless People,* York: Centre for Housing Policy, University of York.

Bines, W., Kemp, P.A., Pleace, N. and Radley, C. (1993) *Managing Social Housing,* London: HMSO.

Black, D., Whitehead, M., Townsend, P. and Davidson, N. (1992) *Inequalities in Health: the Black Report* (rev. edn), London: Penguin.

Boddy, M. (1980) *The Building Societies,* London: Macmillan.

Bourdieu, P. (1984) *Distinction: a Social Critique of the Judgement of Taste,* London: Routledge.

—— (1990) *In Other Words,* Cambridge: Polity Press.

Bradshaw, J. (1972) 'A taxonomy of social need', in G. McLachlan (ed.) *Problems and Progress in Medical Care,* Oxford: Nuffield Provincial Hospital Trust.

Bramley, G. (1993) 'Explaining the incidence of statutory homelessness in England', *Housing Studies* 8(2): 128–47.

British Association of Social Work (BASW)(1985) *Housing and Social Work,* Birmingham: BASW.

Burrows, R. (1996) 'Cyberpunk as social theory: William Gibson and the sociological imagination', in S. Westwood and J. Williams (eds) *Imagining Cities,* London: Routledge.

—— (1997) 'Virtual culture, urban social polarisation and social science fiction', in B. Loader (ed.) *The Governance of Cyberspace,* London: Routledge.

Butler, K., Carlisle, B. and Lloyd, R. (1994) *Homelessness in the 1990s: Local Authority Practice,* London: Shelter.

Cain, M. (1986) 'Who loses out on Paradise Island? The case of defendant debtors in county court', in I. Ramsay (ed.) *Debtors and Creditors,* Abingdon: Professional Books.

Canaan, J. (1996) 'One thing leads to another: drinking, fighting and working-class masculinities', in M. MacAnGhaill (ed.) *Understanding Masculinities,* Buckingham: Open University Press.

Canter, D., Drake, M., Littler, T., Moore, J., Stockley, D. and Ball, J. (1990) *The Faces of Homelessness in London. Interim Report to the Salvation Army*, Department of Psychology: University of Surrey.

Carey, S. (1995) *Private Renting in England*, London: HMSO.

Carlen, P. (1996) *Jigsaw: a Political Criminology of Youth Homelessness*, Buckingham: Open University Press.

Carlisle, J. (1996) *The Housing Needs of Ex-Prisoners*, Centre for Housing Policy Research Report, York: University of York.

Carter, J. (ed.) (1997) *Postmodernity and the Fragmentation of Welfare*, London: Routledge.

Caton, C.M. (ed.) (1990) *Homeless in America*, Oxford: Oxford University Press.

Centrepoint (1988) *No Way Home*, London: Centrepoint.

Chatrik, B. (1994) *Foyers: a Home and a Job?* London: Youthaid.

Citizens' Advice Scotland (1994) *No Help, No Home*, Edinburgh: Citizens' Advice Scotland.

Citron, K.M., Southern, A. and Dixon, M. (1995) *Out of the Shadows: Detecting and Treating Tuberculosis among Single Homeless People*, London: CRISIS.

Clapham, D., Kemp, P.A. and Smith, S. (1990) *Housing and Social Policy*, Basingstoke: Macmillan.

Clapham, D., Munro, M. and Kay, H. (1994) *A Wider Choice: Revenue Funding Mechanisms for Housing and Community Care.* York: Joseph Rowntree Foundation.

Cohen C.I. and Thompson, K.S. (1992) 'Homeless mentally ill or mentally ill homeless', *American Journal of Psychiatry* 149(6): 816–21.

Coles, B. (1995) *Youth and Social Policy*, London: UCL Press.

Concato, J. and Rom, W.N. (1994) 'Endemic tuberculosis among homeless men in New York City', *Archives of Internal Medicine* 154: 2069–73.

Connelly, J. and Crown, J. (eds) (1994) *Homelessness and Ill Health*, London: Royal College of Physicians.

Connelly, J., Kelleher, C., Morton, S., St George, D. and Roderick, P. (1992) *Housing or Homelessness: a Public Health Perspective,* London: Faculty of Public Health.

Conservative Party (1992) *Election Manifesto,* London: Conservative Central Office.

Conway, J. and Kemp, P.A. (1985) *Bed and Breakfast: Slum Housing of the Eighties*, London: Shelter Housing Aid Centre.

Cooper, R., Watson, L. and Allan, G. (1993) *Shared Living in Supported Housing*, Research carried out by the Department of Sociology and Social Policy, University of Southampton, York: Joseph Rowntree Foundation, Housing Research Findings No. 99.

Council of Mortgage Lenders (CML) (1996) 'Statistics on mortgage arrears and possessions', press release.

Craib, I. (1992) *Anthony Giddens*, London: Routledge.

Craig, T. and Timms, P.W. (1992) 'Out of the wards and onto the streets? Deinstitutionalisation and homelessness in Great Britain', *Journal of Mental Health* 1: 265–75.

CRASH (Construction Industry Relief for the Single Homeless) 1995 and 1996 statistics on the use of winter shelters provided in London, London: Crash.

Crook, A.D.H., Kemp, P.A. and Hughes, J. (1995) *The Supply of Privately Rented Homes: Today and Tomorrow*, York: Joseph Rowntree Foundation.

Crook, J. and Dalgleish, M. (1994) 'Homeless young people into jobs and homes – a study of the foyer pilots', *Employment Gazette* (March).

Dant, T. and Deacon, A. (1989) *Hostels to Homes? The Rehousing of Single Homeless People*, Aldershot: Avebury.

Davies, J., Lle, S. with Deacon, A., Law, I., Kay, H. and Julienne, L. (1996) 'Homeless young black and minority ethnic people in England', Department Working Paper No. 15, School of Sociology and Social Policy, University of Leeds.

Davis, M. (1992) 'Beyond blade runner: urban control – the ecology of fear', Westfield, NJ: Open Magazine Pamphlet Series.

Deacon, A., Vincent, J. and Walker, R. (1995) 'Whose choice, hostels or homes? Policies for single homeless people', *Housing Studies* 10(3): 345–63.

Department for Education and Employment (DfEE)(1995) *TECs Getting Results: Equal Opportunities and Special Training Needs – Tackling Training and Employment Needs of Homeless People (revision)*, London: DfEE.

Department of the Environment (1974) *Homelessness*, DoE/DHSS Circular 18/74, London: HMSO.

—— (1991) *Homelessness Code of Guidance for Local Authorities* (3rd edn), London: HMSO.

—— (1993) *English House Condition Survey: 1991*, London: HMSO.

—— (1994a) 'Access to local authority and housing association tenancies: a consultation paper', London: DoE.

—— (1994b) *Housing Strategies: Guidance for Local Authorities on the Preparation of Housing Strategies*, London: HMSO.

—— (1994c) *Circular 18, February 1994: The Ring Fenced Housing Revenue Account*, London: Department of the Environment.

—— (1995a) *Our Future Homes: Opportunity, Choice, Responsibility*, London: HMSO.

—— (1995b) *An Evaluation of the Department of the Environment's S73 Programme*, Housing Research Summary, 41.

—— (1995c) *Survey of English Housing*, London: HMSO.

—— (1995d) *Information Bulletin: Households and Accomodation under the Homelessness Provisions of the 1985 Housing Act, England*, London: HMSO.

—— (1996) *Information Bulletin: Households Found Accommodation under the Homelessness Provisions of the 1985 Housing Act: England – Statistics for the Second Quarter of 1996*, London: Government Statistical Service.

—— (various) *Quarterly Homelessness Returns*.

Department of the Environment/Department of Health (1993) 'Housing and Community Care', Circular 10/92 and LAC (92) 12, London: HMSO.

Department of the Environment, Department of Health, Welsh Office (1992) *Homelessness Code of Guidance for Local Authorities* (3rd edn), London: HMSO.Department of Health (1993) *Health of the Nation*, London: HMSO.

Department of Health (1993) *Health of the Nation*, London: HMSO.

—— (1994) *Housing and Homelessness: Report of the Community Care Monitoring Special Study, October 1993.* (April), London: Department of Health.

Department of Health, Community Care Support Force (1993) *Community Care Services for Homeless People: Managing a Different Sort of Market*, London: Department of Health.

Department of Health and Social Security (1974) Local Authority Circular 13/74, London: HMSO.

Department of Social Security (1992) *Households with Below Half Average Incomes*, London: HMSO.

—— (1995) Statutory Instrument 1644, London: HMSO.

Digby, P.W. (1976) *Hostels and Lodgings for Single People*, OPCS, London: HMSO.

Dillon, L.J. (1991) in *First National Bank plc* v. *Syed,* 2 A11 ER 250 at 251.

Doling, J., Karn, V. and Stafford, B. (1984) 'Mortgage arrears and variability in county court decisions', Working Paper No. 95, Centre for Urban and Regional Research, Birmingham.

Doling, J., Stafford, B. and Ford, J. (1989) *The Property Owing Democracy*, Aldershot: Avebury.

Dominian, J. (1991) *Marital Breakdown and the Health of the Nation*, London: One plus One.

Donnison, D. and Ungerson, C. (1982) *Housing Policy*, London: Penguin Books.

Dorling, D. and Cornford, J. (1995) 'Who has negative equity? How house price falls in Britain have affected different groups of home buyers', *Housing Studies* 10(2): 151–78.

Drake, M. (1985) 'The housing of homeless single people', *Housing Review* 3: 34.

Drake, M. and Biebuych, T. (1977) *Policy and Provision for the Single Homeless: a Position Paper*, London: A Report to the Personal Social Services Council.

Drake, M., O'Brien, M. and Biebuych, T. (1982) *Single and Homeless*, Department of the Environment, London: HMSO.

Elam, G. (1992) *Survey of Admissions to London Resettlement Units*, Department of Social Security, Research Report No.12, London: HMSO.

Evans, A. (1991) *Alternatives to Bed and Breakfast: Temporary Housing Solutions for Homeless People*, London: National Housing and Town Planning Council, supported by Joseph Rowntree Foundation.

—— (1996) *'We Don't Choose to be Homeless . . .'*, Report of the National Inquiry into Preventing Youth Homelessness, London: Campaign for the Homeless and Roofless.

Evans, A. and Duncan, S. (1988) *Responding to Homelessness: Local Authority Policy and Practice*, London: HMSO.

Finer, S.E. (1952) *The Life and Times of Sir Edwin Chadwick*, London: Methuen.

Fisher, K. and Collins, J. (eds) (1993) *Homelessness, Health Care and Welfare Provision*, London: Routledge.
Fisher, N., Turner, S.W., Pugh, R. and Taylor, C. (1994) 'Estimating numbers of homeless people and homeless mentally ill people in North East Westminster by using capture-recapture analysis', *British Medical Journal* 308: 816–19.
Ford, J. (1989–96) Annual reports on arrears and possessions, *Roof* (June/July).
—— (1993) 'Mortgage possession', *Housing Studies* 8(4): 227–40.
—— (1994) *Problematic Home Ownership,* Loughborough: Loughborough University and Joseph Rowntree Foundation.
—— (1995) *Which Way Out? Borrowers in Long Term Arrears*, London: Shelter.
Ford, J. and Kempson, E. (1997a) *Bridging the Gap: Safety Nets for Mortgage Borrowers*, University of York: Centre for Housing Policy.
Ford, J., Kempson, E. and Wilson, M. (1995) *Mortgage Arrears and Possessions: Perspectives from Borrowers, Lenders and the Courts*, London: HMSO.
Ford, J., Quilgars, D., Burrows, R. and Pleace, N. (1997b) *The Housing Needs of Young People in Rural Areas*, London: Rural Development Commission.
Ford, J. and Wilcox, S. (1992) *Mortgage Arrears: an Evaluation of the Initiatives*, York: Joseph Rowntree Foundation.
—— (1994) *Affordable Housing, Low Income and the Flexible Labour Market*, London: NFHA.
—— (1996) 'Owner occupation, employment and welfare: changing relationships and growing exclusion?' Paper presented to Housing Studies Association Conference, September, University of Birmingham.
Forrest, R., Kennett, P. and Leather, P. (1994) *Home Owners in Negative Equity*, Bristol: School for Advanced Urban Studies.
Forrest, R. and Murie, A. (1988) *Selling the Welfare State: the Privatisation of Public Housing*, London: Routledge.
—— (1994) 'Home ownership in recession', *Housing Studies* 9(1): 55–74.
Foster, S. (1992) *Mortgage Rescue: What Does It Add Up To?* London: Shelter.
Foucault, M. (1979) *Discipline and Punish*, Harmondsworth: Penguin.
Fuchs, H.E. (1988) *Becoming an Ex: the Process of Role Exit*, Chicago: University of Chicago Press.
Garside, P., Grimshaw, R. and Ward, F. (1990) *No Place Like Home: the Hostels Experience*, Department of the Environment, London: HMSO.
Gauldie, E. (1974) *Cruel Habitations*, London: George Allen & Unwin.
Geddes J., Newton, R., Young, G., Bailey, S., Freeman, C. and Priest, R. (1994) 'Comparison of the prevalence of schizophrenia among residents of hostels for homeless people in 1966 and 1992', *British Medical Journal* 308: 816–19.
Gibbins, J. (ed.) (1989) *Contemporary Political Culture: Politics in a Postmodern Age*, London: Sage.
Giddens, A. (1979) *Central Problems in Social Theory*, London: Macmillan.
—— (1984) *The Constitution of Society: Outline of the Theory of Structuration*, Cambridge: Polity Press.

—— (1991) *Modernity and Self Identity*, Cambridge: Polity Press.
Glastonbury, B. (1971) *Homeless Near a Thousand Homes*, London: George Allen & Unwin.
GLC/LBA (1981) *Hostels for the Single Homeless in London*, London: London Boroughs Association.
Goffman, E. (1961) *Asylums*, London: Penguin Books.
Graham, H. (1984) *Women, Health and the Family*, Brighton: Wheatsheaf Books.
Great Chapel Street (1995) *Annual Report,* London: Great Chapel Street Medical Centre.
Green, H. and Hansbro, J. (1995) *Housing in England 1993/4: a Report of the 1993/4 Survey of English Housing*, London: HMSO.
Green, H., Thomas, M., Iles, N. and Down, D. (1996) *Housing in England 1994/5: a Report of the 1994/5 Survey of English Housing*, London: HMSO.
Greve, J. (1964) *London's Homeless*, London: The Codicote Press.
—— (1991) *Homelessness in Britain*, York: Joseph Rowntree Foundation.
Greve, J., Page, D. and Greve, S. (1971) *Homelessness in London*, Edinburgh: Scottish Academic Press.
Griffith, A. (1993) 'A shrinking safety net? An examination of the payment of mortgage interest within the income support system', Unpublished LLM thesis, University of Leicester.
Grigsby, C., Baumann, D., Gregorich, S.E. and Roberts-Gray, C. (1990) 'Disaffiliation to entrenchment: a model of understanding homelessness', *Journal of Social Issues* 46: 141–56.
Gurney, C. (1990) 'The meaning of home in the decade of owner-occupation: towards an experiential perspective', Working Paper 88, School of Advanced Urban Studies: University of Bristol.
Gutterman, D. (1994) 'Postmodernism and the interrogation of masculinity', in H. Brod and M. Kaufman (eds) *Theorizing Masculinities*, London: Sage.
HACAS (1995) *Housing Association Involvement in Mortgage Rescue: an Evaluation of the Initiatives*, London: Housing Corporation.
Hagell, A., Newburn, T. and Rowlingson, K. (1995) *Financial Difficulties on Release from Prison*, London: Policy Studies Institute.
Harker, M., Kilgallon, B., Palmer, J. and Tickell, C. (1996) *Making Connections: Policy and Governance for Community Care*, London: Special Needs Housing Association Group.
Harrison, M., Chandler, R. and Green, G. (1991) *Hostels in London: a Statistical Overview*, London: Resource Information Service.
Health Visitors' Association (HVA) and General Medical Services Committee (GMSC)(1988) *Homeless Families and their Health*, London: HVA and GMSC.
Herr, M. (1977) *Dispatches*, London: Picador.
Hewitt, M. (1992) *Welfare, Ideology and Need: Developing Perspectives on the Welfare State*, Hemel Hempstead: Harvester Wheatsheaf.
Hinton, T. (1992) *Health and Homelessness in Hackney*, London: The Medical Campaign Project.
—— (1994) *Battling through the Barriers: a Study of Single Homelessness in Newham and Access to Health Care*, London: Health Action for Homeless People and East London and the City FHSA.

Hockey, J. (1986) *Squaddies, Portrait of a Subculture*, Exeter: Exeter University Press.

Hogarth, T., Elias, P. and Ford, J. (1996) *Mortgages, Families and Jobs*, Warwick: Institute for Employment Research.

Holmans, A. (1995) *Housing Demand and Need in England 1991–2011*, York: Joseph Rowntree Foundation.

Home Office (1995) *Prison Statistics, England and Wales, 1991*, Cm 2893, London: HMSO.

House of Commons Health Committee (1994) *Better Off in the Community: the Care of People who are Seriously Mentally Ill 1993/4*, 102, paras 51 and 58.

Housing Corporation (1995) *Housing Associations in 1994*, London: Housing Corporation.

Huby, M. and Dix, G. (1992) *Evaluating the Social Fund*, London: HMSO.

Hughes, D. and Lowe, S. (1995) *Social Housing Law and Policy*, London: Butterworths.

Hutson, S. and Liddiard, M. (1994) *Youth Homelessness: the Construction of a Social Issue*, London: Macmillan.

Jenkins, R. (1992) *Pierre Bourdieu*, London: Routledge.

Jenn, M. (1993) *Rent Guarantee Scheme Handbook: Housing Homeless People in the Private Rented Sector*, Manchester: National Churches Housing Coalition.

—— (1994) *Rent Guarantee Scheme Handbook: Housing Homeless People in the Private Rented Sector*, Manchester: National Churches Housing Coalition.

Johnson, B., Murie, A., Naumann, L. and Yanetta, A. (1991) *A Typology of Homelessness*, Final Report for Scottish Homes, Edinburgh: Scottish Homes.

Jolly, R. (1996) *Changing Step, from Military to Civilian Life: People in Transition*, London: Brassey's.

Jones, G. (1995) *Leaving Home*, Buckingham: Open University Press.

Jones, H. (1987) *Research Project on the Problem of Single Homelessness in West Yorkshire*, Final Report, University of Leeds: Department of Social Policy and Health Services Studies.

Joseph Rowntree Foundation (1996) 'Inter-agency working for housing, health and social care needs of people in general needs housing', *Housing Research Findings*, 183.

Kay, A. and Legg, C. (1986) *Discharge to the Community: a Review of Housing and Support in London for People Leaving Care*, London: Housing Research Group.

Kemp, P.A. and McLaverty, P. (1995) *Private Tenants and Restrictions in Rent for Housing Benefit*, York: Centre for Housing Policy.

Kemp, P.A., Oldman, C., Rugg, J. and Williams, T. (1994) *The Effect of Benefit on Housing Decisions*, London: HMSO.

Kemp, P.A. and Rhodes, D. (1994) *The Lower End of the Private Rented Sector: a Glasgow Case Study*, Edinburgh: Scottish Homes.

Keyes, S. and Kennedy, M. (1992) *Sick to Death of Homelessness*, London: CRISIS.

Knight, M. (ed.) (1994) *Housing, Homelessness and Health*, Working Group Report: Nuffield Provincial Hospitals Trust for the Standing Conference on Public Health.

Laing, R. (1990) *The Divided Self, an Existential Study in Sanity and Madness*, London: Penguin.

Lash, S. and Urry, J. (1994) *Economies of Signs and Space*, London: Sage.

Lissauer, T., Richman, S., Tempia, M., Jenkins, S., Taylor, B. and Spencer, N.J (1993) 'Influence of homelessness on acute admissions to hospital', *Archives of Disease in Childhood* 93(4): 423–9.

London Research Centre (LRC)(1991) *The Local Impact of Private Sector Leasing*, London: LRC.

Lord Chancellor's Department (LCD)(1991) *Mortgage Possession Statistics*, London: Lord Chancellor's Department.

—— (1996) *Mortgage Possession Statistics*, London: Lord Chancellor's Department.

Luba, J., Madge, N. and McConnell, P. (1993) *Defending Possession Proceedings*, 3rd edn, London: Legal Action Group.

Lupton, C. (1985) *Moving Out: Older Teenagers Leaving Residential Care*, Portsmouth: Social Services Research and Intelligence Unit.

McCluskey, J. (1993) *Reassessing Priorities: the Children Act 1989: a New Agenda for Young Homeless People*, London: Campaign for the Homeless and Rooflеss.

—— (1994) *Acting in Isolation: an evaluation of the Effectiveness of the Children Act for Young Homeless People*, London: CHAR.

McIvor, G. and Taylor, M. (1995) *Supported Accommodation for Ex-offenders: Identifying Effective Practice, a Research Report*, The Department of Applied Social Science: University of Stirling.

Maclennan, D. (1994) *A Competitive UK Economy: the Challenge for Housing Policy*, York: Joseph Rowntree Foundation.

Malpass, P. and Murie, A. (1994) *Housing Policy and Practice*, 4th edn, London: Macmillan.

Marshall, M. (1989) 'Collected and neglected: are Oxford hostels for the homeless filling up with disabled psychiatric patients?' *British Medical Journal* 301: 263–6.

Martin, P., Wiles, R., Pratten, B., Gorton, S. and Green, J. (1992) *A User Perspective: Views on London's Acute Health Services*, London: The King's Fund.

Mason, P. (1994) 'The figures that flatter to deceive', *Inside Housing* (30 September), 10–11.

Means, R. (1993) 'Commentary on housing and community care: from rhetoric to reality', *Community Care Management and Planning* 1(5): 147–9.

Means, R. and Smith, R. (1994) *Community Care: Policy and Practice*, London: Macmillan.

Metcalfe, H. and Christie, I. with Crowley-Bainton, T. and Rolfe, E. (1992) *Employment Initiatives for Homeless People: Report of a Study for the Employment Department*, London: Employment Department.

Morgan, D. (1990) 'No more heroes', in L. Jamieson and H. Corr (eds) *State, Private Life and Political Change*, London: Macmillan.

—— (1994) 'Theater of war: combat, the military, and masculinities', in H. Brod and M. Kaufman (eds) *Theorizing Masculinities*, London: Sage.

Morris, J. (1995) *Housing and Floating Support: a Review*, York Publishing Services.

Mullins, D. (1991) *Housing Services for Homeless People*, Performance Standards Series, Coventry: Institute of Housing.

Munro, M. and Madigan, R. (1993) 'Privacy in the private sphere', *Housing Studies* 8(1): 29–45.

Murphy, A. (1994) 'Analysis of family expenditure survey' (cited in Ford *et al.* 1995), *Mortgage Arrears and Possessions: Perspectives from Borrowers, Lenders and the Courts*, London: HMSO.

NACRO (1982) *Supported Housing Projects for Single People*, London: NACRO.

National Association of Citizens' Advice Bureaux (NACAB) (1995) *Dispossessed*, London: NACAB.

National Consumer Council (1992) *Mortgage Arrears: Services to Borrowers in Debt*, London: National Consumer Council.

National Health Service Advisory Service (1995) *A Place in Mind: Commissioning and Providing Mental Health Services for People who are Homeless*, London: HMSO.

Neale, J. (1995) *The Role of Supported Hostel Accommodation in Meeting the Needs of Homeless People*. DPhil. thesis: University of York.

—— (1996) *Supported Hostels for Homeless People: a Review*, Centre for Housing Policy Research Report, York: University of York.

—— (1997) 'Homelessness and theory reconsidered', *Housing Studies* 12(1): 47–61.

NFHA and SITRA (1991) *Staffing and Employment: Issues in Hostels and Shared Housing*, London: National Federation of Housing Associations.

Niner, P. (1989) *Homelessness in Nine Local Authorities: Case Studies of Policy and Practice*, London: HMSO.

Nixon, J. and Hunter, C. (1996) 'Better a public tenant than a private borrower be: the possession process and threat of eviction', Paper presented to the Housing Studies Association Conference, Birmingham (September).

Nixon, J., Smith, Y., Wishart, B. and Hunter, C. (1996) *Housing Cases in the County Courts*, School of Urban and Regional Studies, Sheffield Hallam University.

Nocon, A. (1994) *Collaboration in Community Care in the 1990s*, Sunderland: Business Education Publisher.

O'Brien, S. (1993) 'Morale and the inner life in the Armed Forces', *Therapeutic Communities* 14(4): 285–95.

Office of Population Censuses and Surveys (OPCS) (1991) *1991 Census: Preliminary Report for England and Wales, Supplementary Monitor on People Sleeping Rough*, London: HMSO.

—— (1994) *1991 Census, Key Statistics for Local Authorities*, London: HMSO.

—— (1995) *General Household Survey*, London: HMSO.

Oldman, C. (1988) 'More than bricks and mortar', *Housing* (June/July): 13–14.

Oldman, C., Quilgars, D. and Oldfield, N. (1996) *Housing Benefit and Services: an Examination of Eligible Housing Costs*, London: HMSO.

Pahl, J. (1982) *The Allocation of Money and the Structuring of Inequality within Marriage*, Canterbury: Health Services Research Unit, University of Kent.

Pascall, G. (1991) *Social Policy: a Feminist Analysis*, London and New York: Routledge.

Paylor, I. (1992) *Homelessness and Ex-offenders: a Case for Reform*, Norwich, University of East Anglia: Social Work Monographs.

Pinch, H. (1993) 'The barriers to homeless people accessing community care', *Community Care Planning and Management* 1(5): 131–6.

Pleace, N. (1995) *Housing Vulnerable Single Homeless People*, York: Centre for Housing Policy.

Pleace, N. and Quilgars, D. (1996) *Health and Homelessness in London: a Review*, London: The King's Fund.

Prescott-Clarke, P., Clemens, S. and Park, A. (1994) *Routes in Local Authority Housing: a New Study of Local Authority Waiting Lists and New Tenancies*, London: HMSO.

Pringle, R. and Watson, S. (1992) 'Women's interests and the post-structuralist state', in M. Barrett and A. Phillips (eds) *Destabilizing Theory: Contemporary Feminist Debates*, Cambridge: Polity Press in association with Basil Blackwell Publishers, Oxford.

Prior, C. (1994) 'Climb the mountain of community care', *Inside Housing* (September): 14–15.

Prior, L. (1995) 'Chance and modernity' in R. Bunton, S. Nettleton and R. Burrows (eds) *The Sociology of Health Promotion*, London: Routledge.

Ramazanoğlu, C. (1989) *Feminism and the Contradictions of Oppression*, London and New York: Routledge.

Randall, G. and Brown, S. (1993) *The Rough Sleepers Initiative: an Evaluation*, London: HMSO.

—— (1994) *Falling Out, a Research Study of Homeless Ex-Service People*, London: Crisis.

—— (1996) *Street to Home*, London: HMSO.

Richards, J. (1993) 'A new sense of duty', *Roof* (September/October): 34–7.

Roberts, K. (1995) *Youth and Employment in Modern Britain*, London: Oxford University Press.

Rock, P. (1973) *Making People Pay*, London: Routledge.

Rosenheck, R. and Fontana, A. (1994) 'A model of homelessness among male veterans of the Vietnam War generation', *Hospital and Community Psychiatry* 151(9): 421–7.

Royal College of Physicians (1994) *Homelessness and Ill Health: Report of a Working Party of the Royal College of Physicians*, London: Royal College of Physicians.

Rugg, J. (1996) *Opening Doors: Helping People on Low Income Secure Private Rented Accommodation*, York: Centre for Housing Policy.

Rugg, J., Rhodes, D. and Willington, S. (1995) 'Students in the private rented sector in York', Unpublished report to the Bursar's Office, University of York.

Saunders, H. (1991) 'Pulling up the ladder', *Roof* (September/October): 9.

Saunders, P. and Williams, P. (1988) 'The constitution of the home: towards a research agenda', *Housing Studies* 3(2): 81–93.

Scheuer, M.A., Black, M., Victor, C., Benezeval, M., Gill, M. and Judge, K. (1991) *Homelessness and the Utilisation of Acute Hospital Services in London*, London: The King's Fund.

Scott, J. (1993) 'Homelessness and mental illness', *British Journal of Psychiatry* 162 (March): 314–24.

Scottish Homes (1996) *Consumer Preferences in Housing*, Edinburgh: Scottish Homes.

Segal, L. (1987) *Is the Future Female? Troubled Thoughts on Contemporary Feminism*, London: Virago Press Ltd.

Shanks, N. and Smith, S. (1992) 'Public policy and the health of homeless people', *Policy and Politics* (20)1: 35–46.

Shanks, P. (1988) 'Medical morbidity of the homeless', *Journal of Epidemiology and Health* 42: 183–6.

Shelter (1992) *The Foyer Project: a Collection of Background Papers, Part I and Part II*, London: Shelter.

—— (1996) *Not an Answer – Private Renting for Homeless Households*, London: Shelter.

Smith, G., Noble, M., Smith, S. and Munby, T. (1991) *The Impact of the 1989 Social Security Changes on Hostel and Board and Lodging Claimants*, Research study funded by the Joseph Rowntree Foundation, Oxford: Oxford University, Department of Applied Social Studies and Social Research.

Smith, N., Wright, C. and Dawson, T. (1992) *Customer Perceptions of Resettlement Units*, Department of Social Security, Research Report No.11, London: HMSO.

Snow, D.A. and Anderson, L. (1987) 'Identity work among the homeless: the verbal construction and avowal of personal identities', *American Journal of Sociology* 92: 1336–71.

Social Security Advisory Committee (1992) *The Social Fund: a New Structure*, London: HMSO.

Somerville, P. (1992) 'Homelessness and the meaning of home: rooflessness or rootlessness?' *International Journal of Urban and Regional Research*, 16(4): 529–39.

Spaull, S. and Rowe, S. (1992) *Silt-up or Move-on? Housing London's Single Homeless*, London: SHiL.

Standing Conference on Public Health (1994) *Housing, Homelessness and Public Health*, London: Nuffield Provincial Hospitals Trust.

Stern, R., Brecht, M., Shuler, P. and Woo, M. (1989) *From the Margins to the Mainstream: Collaboration in Planning Services with Single Homeless People*, London: West Lambeth Health Authority.

Stewart, A. (1996) *Rethinking Housing Law,* London: Sweet & Maxwell.

Sullivan, O. (1986) 'Housing movements of the divorced and seperated', *Housing Studies* 1(1): 35–48.

Taylor, K. and Bloor, K. (1994) *Health Care, Health Promotion and the Future of General Practice*, London: The Nuffield Provincial Hospitals Trust and the Royal Society of Medicine Press.

Taylor, L. and Cohen, S. (1992) *Escape Attempts, the Theory and Practice of Resistance to Everyday Life* (2nd edn), London: Routledge.

Terry, R. (1996) *Changing Housing Markets: the Case for Flexible Tenure and Flexible Mortgages*, London: National Federation of Housing Associations.

Thomas, A. and Niner, P. (1989) *Living in Temporary Accommodation: a Survey of Homeless People*, Department of the Environment, London: HMSO.

Tilt, A. and Denford, S. (1986) *The Camberwell Replacement Scheme: Experiences of the First Three Years*, London: DHSS.

Timms, P. and Fry, A. (1989) 'Homelessness and mental illness', *Health Trends* 21: 70–1.

Townsend, P. (1964) *The Last Refuge*, London: Routledge & Kegan Paul.

Tunnard, J. (1976) *No Father No Home? A Study of 30 Fatherless Families in Mortgaged Homes,* London: Child Poverty Action Group.

Victor, C. (1992) 'Health status of the temporarily homeless population and residents of North West Thames region', *British Medical Journal* 305: 387–91.

Victor, C.R., Connelly, J., Roderick, P. and Cohen, C. (1989) 'Use of hospital services by homeless families in an inner London district', *British Medical Journal* 229: 725–7.

Vincent, J., Deacon, A. and Walker, R. (1993) *Security, Variety and Glorious Uncertainty: the Experiences of ex-Alvaston Resettlement Unit Residents*, Loughborough: Centre for Research in Social Policy, University of Loughborough.

—— (1995) *Homeless Single Men: Roads to Resettlement?* Aldershot: Avebury.

Vredevoe, J., Brecht, D., Shuler, P. and Woo, M. (1992) 'Risk factors for disease in a homeless population', *Public Health Nursing* 9(4): 263–9.

Wacquant, L. (1995) 'Pugs at work: bodily capital and bodily labour among professional boxers', *Body and Society* 1(1): 65–79.

Walby, S. (1992) 'Post-post modernism? Theorizing social complexity', in M. Barrett and A. Phillips (eds) *Destabilizing Theory: Contemporary Feminist Debates*, Cambridge: Polity Press in association with Basil Blackwell Publishers, Oxford.

Walker, R., Vincent, J. and Deacon, A. (1993) *The Effects of Closing the Resettlement Units*, Research carried out by the Centre for Research in Social Policy, Department of Social Sciences, Loughborough University of Technology and the University of Leeds, York: Joseph Rowntree Foundation, Housing Research Findings No. 98.

Watchman, P. and Robson, P. (1989) *Homelessness and the Law in Britain*, Glasgow: Planning Exchange.

Watson, L. and Cooper, R. (1992) *Housing with Care: Supported Housing and Housing Associations*, York: Joseph Rowntree Foundation.

Watson, S. (1984) 'Definitions of homelessness: a feminist perspective', *Critical Social Policy* 11 (Winter): 60–72.

—— (1986) 'Women and housing or feminist housing analysis?' *Housing Studies* (January): 1–10.

—— (1987) 'Ideas of the family in the development of housing form', in M. Loney (ed.) *The State or the Market*, London: Sage.

—— (1988) *Accommodating Inequality: Gender and Housing*, Sydney: Allen & Unwin.

Watson, S. and Austerberry, H. (1986) *Housing and Homelessness: a Feminist Perspective*, London: Routledge & Kegan Paul.

Webb, S. and Wilcox, S. (1991) *Time for Mortgage Benefits*, York: Joseph Rowntree Foundation.

Weedon, C. (1987) *Feminist Practice and Poststructuralist Theory*, Oxford: Basil Blackwell.

Wenzel, S., Gelberg, L., Bakhtiar, L., Caskey, N., Hardie, E., Redford, C. and Sadler, N. (1993) 'Indicators of chronic homelessness among veterans', *Hospital and Community Psychiatry* 44(12): 1172–6.

White, A., Nicholaas, G., Foster, K., Brown, F. and Carley, S. (1993) *Health Survey for England*, London: HMSO.

Wilcox, S. (1996) *Housing Review 1996/97*, York: Joseph Rowntree Foundation.

Wilcox, S. and Sutherland, H. (1997) *Securing Home Ownership*, London: Council of Mortgage Lenders.

Wilcox, S. and Williams, P. (1996) *Mortgage Arrears: Lessons from the Recession*, London: Council of Mortgage Lenders.

Wilkinson, R. (1996) *Unhealthy Societies*, London: Routledge.

Willett, T. (1990) *Canada's Militia, a Heritage at Risk*, Canada: Conference of Defence Associations.

Williams, F. (1989) *Social Policy: a Critical Introduction; Issues of Race, Gender and Class*, Cambridge: Polity Press, in association with Blackwell Publishers, Oxford.

Wilson, E. (1977) *Women and the Welfare State*, London: Tavistock.

Winkleby, M.A. and White, R. (1992) 'Homeless adults without apparent medical and psychiatric impairment – the onset of morbidity over time', *Hospital and Community Psychiatry* 43(10): 1017–33.

Wolf, L.C. (1990) 'Homeless women', in C.M. Caton (ed.) *Homeless in America*, Oxford: Oxford University Press.

Yamanaka, K., Kondo, T. and Miyao, M. (1994) 'Tuberculosis among the homeless people of Nagoya, Japan', *Respiratory Medicine* 88(10): 763–9.

Ziefert, M. and Brown, K.S. (1991) 'Skill building for effective intervention with homeless families', *The Journal of Contemporary Human Services* 212: 212–19.

Zolopa, A.R., Hahn, J.A., Gorter, R., Miranda, J., Wlodarczyk, D., Peterson, J., Pilote, L. and Moss, A.R. (1994) 'HIV and tuberculosis infection in San Franciso homeless adults', *Journal of the American Medical Association* 272(6): 455–61.

Index